Living WOW Now

Thriving in a SAD World

CallyRae Stone

ISBN: 979-8-9926309-0-9

DEDICATION

To Mikayla,

Thank you for keeping me on track for my deadlines and ambitions. May you always remember who you were born to be and live true to your nature. Life is an adventure and I know no one who demonstrates and embraces that more than you!

My hope is that your generation will recognize the thriving power of Living WOW and step away from surviving the toxic SAD life.

You are the hope of the future.

CONTENTS

ACKNOWLEDGMENTS

A special thank you to Marcie, Brandi, and Jeri who provided feedback and editing with perspective and attention to detail that I lack.

Thank you to my family who have been the guinea pigs for all things Living WOW and keep the eye rolling to a minimum when I have a new epiphany.

Finally, to acknowledge my Father in Heaven as the ultimate authority and Source of wisdom for thriving. I am eternally gratefully for the inspiration and guidance given to me in creating the Living WOW Lifestyle and Framework.

Introduction

Do you sometimes wonder what happened to your life? Whose body is this anyway? Do you feel deep down that there is more for you than *this*? If so…here is your answer! Come sit with me as we journey to thriving in the most miraculous vehicle you didn't even realize you had access to.

As we begin, I'm going to look back a bit, and then cast a vision forward to give you context of WOW. Where we are and what's coming.

In the spring of 2021, I was in the middle of extensive travel and finishing up Transformation 2.0. I had completely fallen into the chaos, fear, scarcity, and isolation that had characterized our society during the pandemic.

It took me all of four months to regress into the autopilot of my pre-transformation lifestyle. I had left behind my daily routines and habits and recognized pain and autoimmune flares that I had not experienced for 10 years. After realizing that I was once again surviving with my autoimmune diseases, I made the decision.

Feeling literally like I had been transported back in time 12 years; I made the choice to once again take back my life. More specifically, my lifestyle. I knew that I had transformed my health with lifestyle choices once, I could do it again.

In the fall of 2020, I set out on transformation 2.0. I could no longer deal with the pain, flares, exhaustion, depression, fear, and hopelessness.

So, in these three steps, this is what happened:

Number one, I set the intention. I knew that I had successfully transformed from surviving to thriving before, so logic would tell me that I could do it again. I literally reread my own book; *8 Lessons Lupus*

Taught Me: From Surviving to Thriving with Autoimmune Diseases! That put me in the mindset and gave me the hope that I could do it again.

Number two, I then put into action the mechanisms necessary to get back to thriving. I did them through the fall and the winter making sure I had my structure and using the tools that I knew and that I had, but had fallen away from using.

Number three, I reengaged and finished what I started. We were in the middle of a 50-state book tour the year I turned 50, this was our 50 in 50, to share the message of thriving with autoimmune disease and doing the Change Your Story presentations and book signings.

That's when the shutdown happened and we were, of course, grounded from travel and unable to complete our southern route or the cruise to Alaska. I didn't do any book promotions or speaking, even online, because I just didn't feel like I could share thriving in the middle of a global pandemic.

As spring emerged, and I was making progress with my transformation, I had the realization that it was more important than ever for me to get back out there, whatever it had to look like.

So, we scheduled and rescheduled the remaining states. Rerouting and adjusting as schedules, precautions, closures, and regulations permitted. Finally, in June, it was time to go, and we knew there would be no live presentations or book signings, but we could still share hope. I was feeling about 80 percent with my health and Transformation 2.0.

We completed 24 states in 21 days, and shared informal hope sessions with people all across the country, vlogging every day of the journey. Three weeks later, we had another major travel that was not part of the original 50 in 50. Our family was invited to Mexico to celebrate my daughter's 10th anniversary vow renewal, as well as all of our wedding anniversaries.

I was nervous. I had not traveled internationally since 9/11 and had not flown since COVID, and we had just returned from this exhausting southern route. Would my health hold up? I just didn't know.

Despite the apprehension, I had the commitment to my family and myself, so we went. I came back from Mexico feeling amazing!

I was at least 90%. My flares were at bay, my pain was minimal, and my energy was improving. So finally, three weeks after my return from Mexico, we finished with the trip to Alaska. The final state to finish our 50-state tour. I'm happy to report that as we finished what we started, plus some, I was 100%, I was once again thriving with autoimmune diseases.

It could be done!

That changed everything. Following transformation 2.0 and all of the country we covered, I realized that most things coming at you from the media and social media, from family and friends, are at a rapid rate with a lot of fear, and a lot of survival.

I realized that you not only needed hope, but you needed how.

So, I set out to make a system that was universal, but yet individual. A system simple enough for anyone to learn to be the expert in their body. I came back, not sure if I should write another book or if I should do more individual coaching? How could I make the biggest impact? I felt like the autoimmune community was in worse shape than it was even 12 years earlier when I felt so hopeless.

I finally decided that the answer was in a framework. If I could use a framework that would be universal enough for all of our autoimmune diseases, yet individual enough to answer the lifestyle need, then we would be able to recreate the transformation results.

And that is where Living Wow went from hope and inspiration to a framework to get results. So over the remainder of this book, you will have the opportunity to learn more about the framework and the metaphor that I use to help you understand exactly what is happening in your body and how to understand what it means, and how to facilitate healing so that you can thrive with your autoimmune diseases.

As I have re-transformed and navigated these familiar paths, yet in very different circumstances, I have defined and refined Living WOW to be a simple, effective, and fun framework that you can understand and replicate no matter your situation. I promise it won't hurt and of course your ultimate result is thriving with your autoimmune diseases.

In fact, I'm going to take it one step further based on feedback from podcast listeners of *Living WOW Out Loud* and others who have walked alongside me with the development of the Living WOW Lifestyle. I'm going to say that the Living WOW Lifestyle applies to anyone who wants to thrive. No AI (autoimmune) diagnosis or label is necessary to live a life of thriving.

Of course, the foundation and need for me to build the framework came out of my autoimmune journey, but the resulting comprehensive and universal framework applies to anyone who wants to live their best life and thrive.

Living WOW has become the counter culture narrative to living SAD (Standard American Diet and lifestyle). The autopilot most of us live on as we navigate the chaos and noise of modern culture and technologies.

That is the goal! As I introduce the framework using a metaphor that you can then conceptualize. I'm taking things that are really nebulous and unfamiliar to most people and bringing it to the familiar. It is familiar to you. It is your life.

It is your lifestyle and it doesn't have to be difficult. It doesn't have to be confusing, and it doesn't take an expert to figure out what it means. It may take a guide to teach you how to understand. It may take someone that has been a few miles ahead of you on the journey to make the process a little easier.

That's why I've created the framework to get results. I've moved from knowing that you need hope, to now we have to have the how!

The power is in your body. The power is in your lifestyle. The framework of the Living WOW Lifestyle will help you to identify system failures or maintenance needs. Whether you just need a tune up or a complete systems overhaul, we support you as an individual to get back out on the journey and Living WOW.

So, bring on the Living WOW Lifestyle framework and the journey of life metaphor that follows to take something as complex and individual as your lifestyle and understand it with simple universal experiences and truths.

Following the metaphor and framework, I will get into the application of Living WOW as I introduce you to resources to determine levels of function, needs, tools, and/or providers that may be best equipped to guide you as you step out of the negative health cycle and turn it into a positive health cycle.

What does WOW mean to you?

I've been thinking a lot about WOW lately. What the word means. What experiences make you say WOW. What feelings surround a moment of WOW. Even the letters as an acronym and what they can stand for because Living WOW is the name of the lifestyle program and the framework for thriving with autoimmune disease.

I've been dissecting it, analyzing it, and defining it to bring the mission of Living WOW to you with the characteristics that make it universal, but the details that make it individual to you.

Think about the last time you said, WOW. Do you remember what that was? Do you remember how you felt? Do you remember what was happening?

Mine was this morning as I went for a walk through my neighborhood. The sun was rising as I walked down the sidewalk, noticing the gorgeous spring blossoms decorating the trees. Spring colors were on full display and the birds were chirping a good morning to me. As I walked through the neighborhood, the open sky is lit up with the most beautiful sunrise of pink clouds with orange hues set on a pastel blue backdrop.

"WOW!" I said out loud to myself. That is a gorgeous sunrise. What an amazing way to start the day. I then thanked God for the opportunity to witness this beautiful creation, and enjoyed it as it evolved and eventually dissolved into the daylight.

Upon arriving home, I exclaimed to my husband how gorgeous the sunrise was and how it makes getting up for these early morning walks worth it. If I could do a sunrise walk every morning, it would do so many amazing things for me. I could get in a daily walk for exercise, be in nature, and start the day off right.

We then discussed a time when I did early morning walks with a group of friends in our previous community. I really loved it. Why don't I do that? Why did I stop doing that? How can I start doing it again? What can I do with my schedule or my routines to put that in and get back into a habit that allows me to have these experiences more often?

Have you ever felt that way? That's what's meant by Living WOW.

Living in a way that you are aware of things that bring you joy and make you feel alive. Sharing those moments with those around you and celebrating the wonders of life. Being intentional in the choices you make and how to bring more opportunities to experience WOW moments into your days.

This is what I characterize as thriving, and it's made possible by living WOW. The problem is that I don't always see the sunrise, so I forget how much I love it. I don't want to get up that early. I'm inside working, and I don't get to see that part of the sky. I'm busy with other things, and I miss it.

Basically, I'm on autopilot going through my day and getting things done. I don't make the intentional choice to watch the sun come up, even though I know how much better it would make my days.

Truth is, I forget how much I love it and how much better it would make my days because I've just gotten too far away from it. This is an example of the autopilot that I call the SAD life. The standard American lifestyle of automatic, rush, noise, and busy that distracts us from living our best life.

I easily fall back into SAD because it's exactly that. Easy. Everybody's doing it, whether it's a morning routine, food choices, exercise, sleep, or how we relate to each other. There's a social norm that we fit into and go with the flow.

Have you missed the sunrise too? I use this analogy of the sunrise because it literally happened to me this morning and it's a great reminder to me of the contrast between living SAD and Living WOW.

It's also a great reminder to me of why I'm so passionate about sharing WOW with you because that's the secret to thriving.

Making intentional choices that support the systems of your body to repair and function more optimally is powerful. Living WOW supports a positive health cycle that, once experienced, cannot be ignored.

Living life with energy and awareness that brings joy is available to everyone. But if you're like me, you've lived SAD for so long, you don't believe you could feel WOW. After experiencing my first transformation, I wanted others with autoimmune diseases to understand that you can thrive despite the diagnosis.

In writing the book, *8 Lessons Lupus Taught Me: From Surviving to Thriving with Autoimmune Diseases*, I shared my journey and changed perspective toward my diseases and life as a whole. After tumbling full speed into SAD with the events of 2020 triggering every survival instinct I had, I found myself with pain, weight gain, depression, exhaustion, and flares that I had eliminated years earlier.

I felt like I'd gone back in time 12 years.

What was different this time was my belief. I knew that I could thrive amid difficult times. I knew the process. I had the tools. I knew that it would take a series of perpetual choices and probably a few restarts. I knew it would take time. But I knew it was possible.

So, in the depths of a pandemic and worldwide chaos, I decided to live WOW. I decided to step out of the SAD life that had again consumed my everyday choices. I decided to make a change. What seemed overwhelming and frustrating as I struggled to make order out of chaos slowly started to give glimpses of Living WOW.

Better food choices and supplements kept my immune system strong against the virus battle. Choosing better material for my mind to listen to and focus on kept my mental tracks hopeful. Quieting the chaotic chatter of the world helped me tune into the Spirit and remember who I was born to be and the journey that I'm on.

Nine months later, I had completed what I now refer to as my second transformation. Once again, thriving with autoimmune diseases. I had successfully embraced intentionally Living WOW, and cut the time down from five years for my first transformation to nine months. My second transformation. **WOW**!

After my first transformation, I needed to give hope to those with autoimmune diseases. To not suffer and just survive with a diagnosis and a masking of symptoms that may lead to a cascade of more disease, but instead love your body. Embrace your autoimmune diseases, learn to understand them, and find joy in the journey.

Now, after my second transformation, I'm compelled to give you the framework for Living WOW. To empower you to step out of the SAD and embrace WOW.

Change is scary, and most of us won't run headlong into change because we are comfortable where we are. Even if we aren't comfortable, it's familiar. And, of course, there's that. Moving away from comfort and familiar takes courage, even if we know it's going to be better.

So, just like I came home and told my husband about my sunrise experience, I'm sharing my Living WOW experience with you. Don't you do that? When you eat something delicious, you want to share a bite. When you see something beautiful, you tell someone about it. And when you experience something life changing, you want to have others experience it, too.

Let's Start at the Very Beginning

Autoimmune disease doesn't strike overnight. Although if you live with an autoimmune disease, you know it can feel like you were run over by a freight train overnight and you woke up wondering, what the hell just happened? Generally, when this happens, you run to the doctor because you feel sick.

The doctor looks you over and sends you home with medicine based on your complaints and symptoms. Depending on how many times you've been to the doctor, the severity of your symptoms, or the competency of your doctor, labs may be ordered to support the medication recommendation and look a little deeper.

When was the last time your doctor asked you about your diet, relationships, your work? Education, finances, stress, exercise, or even self-care? Probably never, right? Crazy, because we know that all of these things collectively add up to your health and they're impacting the dis-ease that you're seeking answers for.

Don't get me wrong, I'm not talking about the 'it's all in your head' philosophy that many will put on you because they can't find a physical reason for your incessant pain, rash, stomach pain, fatigue, weight gain, weight loss, (fill in your symptom). Whatever your symptom is that you're going to the doctor for.

You absolutely are experiencing that symptom. Unfortunately, I've known doctors that prescribe antidepressants or anti-anxiety meds when you come in with these complaints because they can't find a physical explanation. Let's just medicate it. You must be depressed.

The questions that they should ask are why? What is the underlying cause of the symptom? How about a whole lifestyle assessment with a look back period more than yesterday? What if you were asked lifestyle questions that included that look back period? Like maybe a week, a month? When did your symptoms start? And not just when did they start, but what was happening in your life at that time?

After asking these questions, what if you were prescribed good mood foods? What if you were prescribed to get outside in nature for an hour a day? What if you were prescribed to move your body doing your favorite activity every day? What if you were prescribed to spend time in an activity with your favorite person? What if you were prescribed to surround yourself with the people that make you the happiest? What if you were prescribed to take a vacation and truly unplug from work, maybe even every three months?

Would these prescriptions solve everything? Yes, maybe, maybe not. Would they have toxic side effects and organ damage, drug interactions, and possibly death? Absolutely not. Would they cover up your symptoms and give you new symptoms making it more difficult to get to the underlying cause of the disease? Nope.

Of course, there are times when it makes sense to visit your doctor. But after more than 25 years in healthcare, and 35 years of learning to understand my own body, you can bet I've learned a few things.

I've learned that medicine is almost always toxic and misused. I've learned that medicine is almost always unnecessary. I've learned that everything we need to heal our bodies has been provided by nature, but we probably don't recognize it or know how to use it.

I've learned that creating an environment to heal is up to me, not my doctor. And I've learned that I don't need permission to be the expert in my own body, but I do need to learn how.

So, I want to start with the low hanging fruit. Just because you know it doesn't mean you do it. We all know that we should be eating healthy food, exercising regularly, and sleeping well. The reality is that few of us actually do because life happens, the SAD life to be exact.

The Standard American Diet and lifestyle is the underlying cause of most diseases, including autoimmune disease, and it's epidemic in our society. What if you decided to stop the SAD and embrace a new life? A WOW life.

What if you ate good mood food? What if you started moving your body by dancing in the kitchen listening to uplifting music while you prepared food that was delicious and nutritious? What if you sat down at the table and ate that good mood food with the people that matter most to you? What if you listened to a podcast or watched a video that inspired you or taught you something new instead of listening to the news or getting caught up in the drama? What if you journaled the wins and desires of the day before you went to bed?

These are what I call the low hanging fruit because you already know what you should be doing. The trick is to stop shoulding on yourself and get into action. Just pick one. Start with today, not tomorrow.

Action is the key, so pick up something that you can do and get a win. That win will lead to the next choice. Do it again, and again, and again. That's basic behavior change, right? Before you know it, you find yourself in a new intentional choice routine, and the guilt and shame of shoulding is behind you.

I'll use good mood food for illustration because it's powerful, simple, and self-reinforcing.

Today, instead of reaching for an energy drink or a sugary snack to pick you up, eat your favorite fruit. The whole fruit, not a canned, dried, or processed form of it. Maybe it's a crispy sweet apple, a juicy orange, an exotic pineapple or mango. Maybe even a superfood of blueberries or pomegranate. It doesn't matter which fruit. Your body will tell you the one that's best for you because you like it and it's available to you.

The nutrient profile in fruit makes it good mood food for anyone, as it gives you a boost of glucose for energy, but metabolizes completely and steadily because of the whole food matrix.

Your cells will thank you because of the vitamins, phytonutrients, minerals, hydration, and glucose that they need to replicate healthy cells. Your gut will thank you because you're supporting a healthy microbiome with prebiotic fiber and encouraging probiotic health and diversity. Your brain will thank you because you just released the chemicals of serotonin by feeding your microbiome a whole fiber rich food.

Are you hesitant to try? Do you find yourself saying, "but fruit is loaded with sugar. I've heard fructose is bad." Well, welcome to SAD! You've been victimized by the Standard American Diet of misinformation because it's far more profitable to addict you to processed 'health' foods that are laden with fake sugar and pseudo ingredients while they manage your medical conditions with prescription medications.

Have you ever tried to overeat whole foods? How many apples can you eat in a sitting? Whole apples. Have you ever tried to eat an entire bowl of blueberries? How about an entire pineapple? Nature tells us the right amount of foods to eat because unlike processed foods, we are not physically able to over-consume whole foods.

So, in addition to the benefits to your cells, gut and brain that I mentioned earlier. You also have the added benefit of not having to count calories, because your body will tell you how much is enough for you.

So that's it. Congratulations. You've just successfully completed an introduction to Living WOW!

You've learned how to choose intentionally to support your body rather than suppress or mask what it's telling you. If you chose to participate in the low hanging fruit exercise, you even learned how to make a choice for good mood food that showers your system with all the goodness it needs and in the amount it needs to give you the lift that supports a WOW life rather than a SAD life.

Now do it again. As you're making those intentional choices, take note of how your body is changing. What feels good? What's the next choice? What's the best choice? As you increase your awareness and begin making intentional WOW choices the momentum increases and the change is easier and easier because it is more and more familiar.

A Simple Metaphor

Do you have a detailed understanding of the complex systems of your body? Do you consider yourself an expert in your body? Do you understand the language of your body and how it speaks to you? Most people I talk with will answer no to these questions.

Most people rely on an outside expert, often a doctor or specialist. As a speech language pathologist, I'm constantly reminding mothers that they know their babies best. They know their routines. They know their behaviors, and even though an infant doesn't speak, they are able to effectively communicate their needs with their mother.

She is able to know whether the cry is a hungry cry or a pain cry. She is able to know how to soothe and care for the baby, not because someone taught her the intricacies of infant communication, but because she has spent time with her baby and speaks her baby's language.

She also knows when something is off even if the baby isn't crying. She's in tune with the baby's nonverbal communication and behaviors and can determine when she needs further help understanding what is happening with the baby. She may call her mom, google it, or go to the doctor. How does a mother know? We all know that babies don't come with an instruction book.

She certainly doesn't ignore it. She can't. It's a nagging certainty that something isn't right and she will usually stick with it until she determines what is off. How does she know? It's instinct. A mother and baby have an instinctual bond and understanding that makes it possible to meet their needs without formal training.

Yes, she may seek help and guidance along the way, but ultimately, she knows her baby best and gives the information to the expert to understand what is off and be able to give guidance.

This is exactly why you are the expert in your body. This understanding of what your body feels like and how it operates is innately programmed into each of us, but we forget it, or even worse, discount or ignore it because we're busy with other things.

This is common with what I refer to as SAD, the Standard American Diet and Lifestyle. We are so busy and distracted that we don't even realize that our bodies are trying to communicate what is needed. When they break down, we get frustrated and angry at them because they're limiting what we can do. We go to the doctor and get medications to treat the pain and symptoms.

I want to introduce you to a simple metaphor that takes complex systems and intricacies of our bodies and helps you tap into your innate understanding of those systems that you likely have never been taught to recognize.

Living WOW Lifestyle Systems

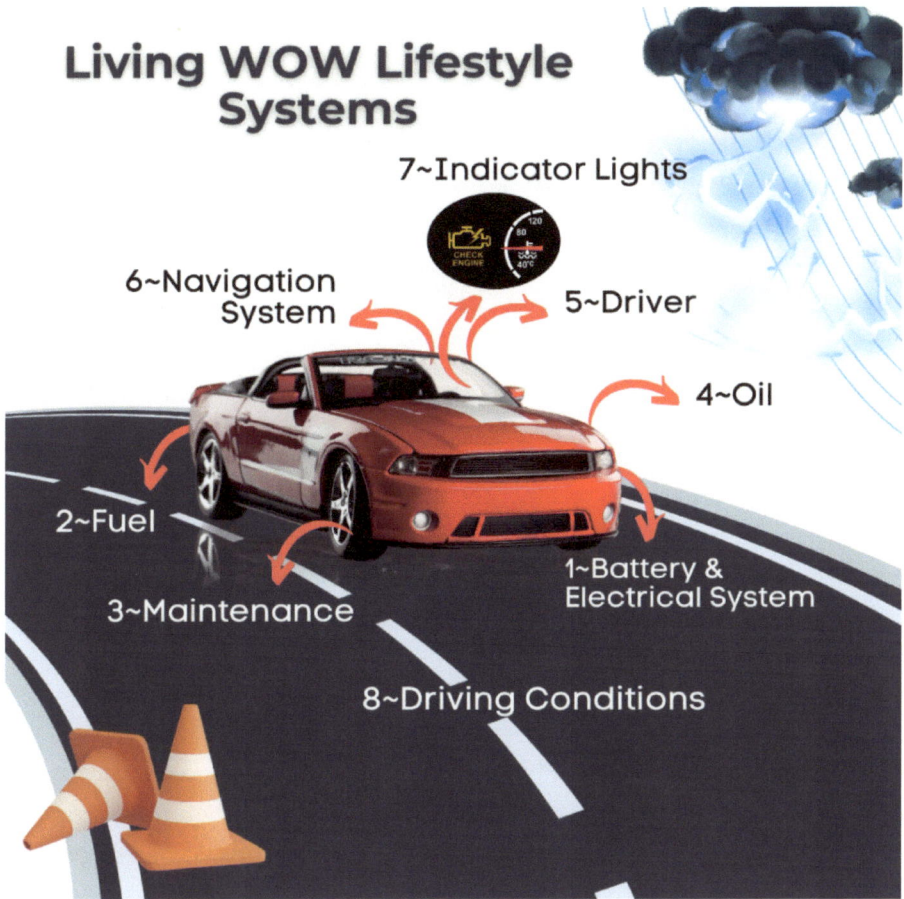

7~Indicator Lights

6~Navigation System

5~Driver

4~Oil

2~Fuel

1~Battery & Electrical System

3~Maintenance

8~Driving Conditions

We each come into this world on a journey. Our journeys look very different for every single one of us, but we are all indeed on a journey called life.

We each have a body with which we navigate this life. Come with me as we explore your body as a vehicle with which we travel through life as a journey. Each vehicle is amazing. It comes perfectly equipped with every special feature you need for your specific journey. Each of our vehicles is individual to our specific journey and the conditions we will encounter along the way.

Of course, all vehicles need power. And that power comes from energy. The battery and electrical systems of your vehicle are not unlike the energetic and nervous systems of your body. If your battery doesn't start, you're dead. And if there's a short in your electrical system, you're not getting very far down the road.

No less important than energy is the fuel, because with an empty tank or the wrong fuel, you are also not getting very far down the road. Of course, food for our bodies is just as important as fuel for our vehicles. Eating the wrong foods is very much like putting diesel in a gas engine. It works great for a diesel engine, but it destroys a gas engine. It's important to know what fuel your vehicle requires as it will affect its function and operation.

Your vehicle requires good quality oil and routine maintenance to continue to operate most efficiently. Not changing the oil, rotating the tires, checking your fluid levels, getting new wipers, tires, or hoses will surely leave you broken down on the side of the road. For our bodies, hydration and supplements help our systems function smoothly. Without systematic and routine self-care, our bodies will experience a similar breakdown.

Each vehicle comes equipped with its own driver. Super cool! But the driver can only do what it's told. The driver is constantly looking for threats and obstacles along the road, making thousands of decisions in minutes, processing like a supercomputer.

The driver's main objective is to get you there alive. That's it. The driver is your mind, and although we think it's smart, it really is just processing what it is told and identifying threats to your survival. The information you are giving your mind to process is what is affecting where you are going and how you are getting there.

The navigation system is actually the smarts of the operation. The navigation system knows the journey and the best routes, the alternative routes and road closures, the delays and the pit stops. Unfortunately, sometimes the navigation system is drowned out by the noise of the vehicle and the road or the environment around it.

Sometimes the navigation system is ignored by the driver because it's not familiar and it deviates from what the driver believes. Our own personal navigation system is our spirit, our eternal intelligence. Our spirit knows the life we were born to live and the capabilities of our bodies. Unfortunately, the spirit within us is quiet and it's often drowned out by the noise of our lifestyles and world.

When we tune into our spirit, we find that all the directions we are seeking are available to us. Sometimes we doubt our spirit because our mind is running on limiting beliefs and incomplete information.

There's a bonus feature! Some vehicles are equipped with special indicator lights that tell you how the systems are functioning. You may get a low fuel warning or a check engine light if a system is failing. Of course, some lights are easier to read than others, but they are telling you exactly where to look for the maintenance and repair.

Ignoring the indicator lights or covering them up is sure to result in a breakdown and possibly even engine failure. Symptoms are the indicator lights of our bodies. Listening to understand what the symptoms are telling us about our systems can give us a shortcut to understanding where we need support and healing. Likewise, ignoring systems or covering them with medications can compound the disease and lead to system failures.

All vehicles come with an owner's manual, but it is often overlooked because we've been taught how to drive and operate the vehicle. Make no mistake that driving the vehicle, any mind can do that, is far different than maintaining it. In order to keep your vehicle in optimal condition while you get where you're going, you'll need to use your owner's manual.

Your vehicle must navigate through all types of weather and driving conditions on your journey. It's not always ideal conditions. Taking a detour or waiting it out may be necessary. Recognize that your vehicle is equipped for your journey, but it may require more maintenance or time to get there. This is not unlike the body getting through this life. We can't control the weather or the conditions around us, but we can control how we prepare and navigate through them.

This is where I come in as the narrator to this metaphor. I guess you could call me a mechanic of sorts. I've been on this journey of life for a bit, and I've been taught about all of these different systems and how to repair them. I recognize that all of our vehicles are different, but there are similarities that when trained to recognize them can be taught and repaired through a lifestyle program.

So, I put it all together in a framework that helps you recognize the warning lights, understand what they mean, and support you with the knowledge and tools to repair the damage. I help guide you to the best mechanic in town.

The 8 Systems

Each of the 8 systems has been put into a framework with a metaphor of a vehicle on a journey to help simplify the very complex systems and help understand abstract systems that we can't see, but we can certainly feel.

The framework to become the expert in your body's 8 systems are:

#1 Your Battery and Electronics = Energy

#2 Your Fuel = Food & Water

#3 Your Maintenance = Self-care & Movement

#4 Your Oil = Supplements

#5 Your Driver = Mind/Intelligence

#6 Your Navigation System = Spirit

#7 Your Indicator Lights = Symptoms

#8 Your Driving Conditions = Environment

In the coming pages, we will deep dive into each of these systems and understand how that metaphor can be applied to a specific system in your body to assess and understand where you may need attention and maintenance.

All of these systems come together to define your own personal Living WOW Lifestyle.

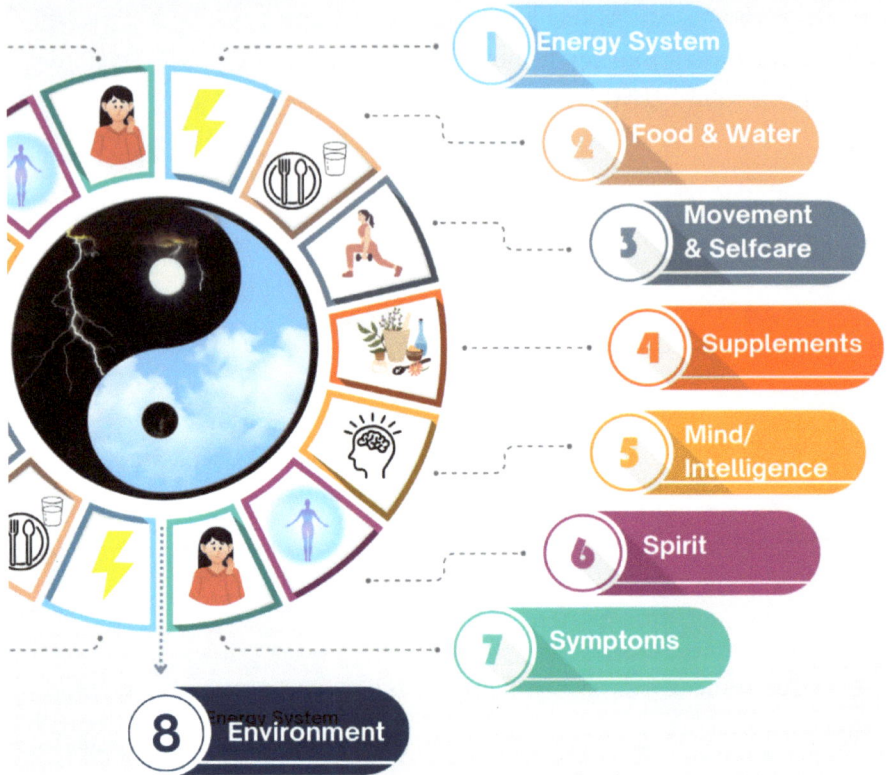

Living WOW Lifestyle Framework

1 Energy System
2 Food & Water
3 Movement & Selfcare
4 Supplements
5 Mind/Intelligence
6 Spirit
7 Symptoms
8 Environment

System 1:
The Electrical System

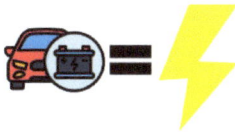

Even though food or fuel was the catalyst for my initial change and is certainly foundational for healing, I really didn't understand energy until a lot farther down my transformation journey. In fact, it was one of the later lessons learned. As I put together the framework for thriving, I realized that energy needs to be addressed first.

The energy system is your batteries and your electronics. If your battery is dead, you're not going anywhere. Even if your battery is not dead, it can impact your function because of poor energy movement. I now understand that all disease starts with some sort of energetic beginning.

Whether this is a block, a disruption, or a leak, it all stems from some sort of energetic foundation. I know when we talk about energy, it can sound very woo woo and nebulous, so some people may avoid the topic. In fact, I think I avoided the topic of energy early on in my transformation because I wasn't aware of the significance and also because I felt like it was off limits.

I was raised in a traditional Christian home and found the power of God to be sacred. To me, things like moving energy or playing with energy were blasphemous or not my place. Maybe that was supernatural or magic. There were a lot of negative connotations of energy work. So for me, I think I avoided it, not really understanding what it was.

When I really realized what it is and how central it is to living, whether you're comfortable with it or not, whether you're aware of it or not, whether you choose to understand it or not. It's still there-much like gravity. So, to understand my beginnings in energy work exploration and understanding of energy fields is in my first book, *8 Lessons Lupus Taught Me: From Surviving to Thriving with Autoimmune Diseases.*

But here, for this purpose, now that we're beyond learning the lessons, it's really for you to understand the practical application. The practical application is that if you understand anything about energy, you understand that it needs an open transmission to be effective. In our bodies, we have different energetic systems, just like we have different physical systems.

I make these basic comparisons to help you understand something you cannot see, but rather feel subjectively. I am not a skilled energy worker, but I do have a basic understanding that enables me to troubleshoot. I am able to provide routine maintenance for my energy systems much like I would my physical systems.

For example, in your body you have a nervous system that is comprised of your brain, spinal cord, cranial nerves, and peripheral nervous system. You also have organs such as your lungs, heart, liver, kidney, stomach, etc. that all have a specific function in your body. You have bones, muscles, and skin that give you the structure of your physical body and protect your body as you interact with your environment.

To me, the correlation to the energy systems is simple, and I'm giving you a basic rundown because really, that's all you need at this level. If, like me, you find interest or want to dive deeper into a specific energy system, you can do that. But for this purpose, it's all about a simple introduction to understanding that it is a foundational consideration to understanding your body.

Your aura is the outer layer of your energy body and is the energy field around you that protects and interacts with your environment. Think of it like your skin. This is the part of your energy system that interacts with other energies when you walk into a room and you might feel calm and attracted to someone or icky and on guard to someone else.

You are experiencing an energy hit or exchange on your aura, much like you experience when you shake hands physically, you feel their skin with your skin. However, your aura is larger and able to feel the energy of others without any physical contact. Similarly, you can damage your aura or pick up undesirable energy, just like you can damage your skin or get dirty.

Your chakras are the seven energetic systems of the body which I compare to the organs because they have a specific location and function much like your organs do. Likewise, each chakra correlates to a physical organ or group of organs.

Recently, my daughter was experiencing severe pain in her ear for a week. She'd been to the doctor, who found no cause for the pain. I asked her if she had been feeling like she wasn't being heard. She looked at me with a strange look and said,

> "Yes! All of this stuff's been going on at work and I feel like my boss isn't listening to me. I'm telling him if we can't meet and talk about a solution, I'm going to have to leave and go work for another office. I don't want to do that because I love the people I work with, but he won't even take the time to listen to what is wrong."

We did some energy clearing techniques and her pain was relieved. The work situation took weeks to resolve, but just recognizing that energy block that had been building up for months and releasing it helped clear the painful physical symptoms that she was experiencing.

Finally, your meridians are the energetic pathways where energy flows, much like your nervous system is the pathway where your nerve impulses are sent and received. You may be familiar with acupuncture or pressure points. These are the pathways and nerve centers that have been mapped out and used in Chinese medicine for healing for centuries.

By releasing a point in the meridian with some sort of physical intervention, such as a needle, pressure, or tapping, you're able to clear a block in the flow of the energy pathway. This block can be due to a physical injury or it can be from an emotional injury.

This was the system that I recognized and understood first because of my background in the brain and the nervous system. I understood the correlation of the meridian maps to the nervous system. You can see the crossover with common practices such as massage and acupuncture.

So to summarize and simplify, your meridians are how your energy flows much like your nervous system. Your chakras are where your energy is managed and used much like your organs, and your aura is the outer layer that is interacting with the environment around you.

Now to relate it back to the framework for becoming the expert in your body and thriving, I want to share a recent experience that helped me understand on a physical level the impact of the energy system. This may help you understand how the energy system can impact physical health in ways that are hard to conceptualize in your body.

My younger daughter has an older car that is her first car. We bought the car from her older sister and knew the history and maintenance of the car. That gave us peace of mind that it was in great condition and should get her through college before she would have to buy a new car.

Almost a year to the day after getting the car, it was shutting down. It was going into limp mode. The shifting would be rough and the car wouldn't accelerate. She would have to get to the side of the road, turn it off, wait a few minutes, and then she'd be able to turn it back on and get where she was going.

This was the symptom, if you will, that got our attention and we couldn't ignore it anymore. She was breaking down on very busy roads and it was taking longer to recover and get to where she was going. It was unsafe so we had to shut it down and park it.

It wasn't like we hadn't done anything. She had a dead battery several months ago, so we had it tested and replaced. We knew that wasn't the issue.

The automatic transmission light was coming on before it would shift funny and act weird. So we had a full transmission service, because it had a lot of miles on it and it was probably due to be serviced. Not a cheap service to have done, but we thought it was necessary because the car wasn't driving properly.

We had a new battery, we had the transmission serviced from top to bottom, and yet the problem continued to persist. So, I talked to a mechanic who said it was probably the TCM unit that tells the transmission how to operate. He offered to run diagnostics and determine whether or not that was the problem.

Of course it was, but because of it being electrical and the age of the car, he would recommend going to a dealer and have it replaced and programmed. Long story short, getting the replacement part and having it reprogrammed by the dealer was going to cost more than the car was worth, and they weren't too motivated to find a part for this old car. I'm sure they would have preferred if I just bought a new one.

Because it was an electrical problem, she was assured by the mechanic that it wasn't damaging the engine to drive it. We limited the use of the car to essential driving only (which is interpreted differently by a 16-year-old than by her parents).

She kept driving and troubleshooting, the stereo went out, the gas mileage was tanking (pun intended), and the driving became more and more unreliable. After talking to the bank about financing options, an abysmal search for a replacement vehicle, and taking it in for an appraisal for a trade in, I learned that the power steering was also going out! We were defeated and frustrated.

This car was in mint condition a year ago, and now it was literally unsafe to drive. I decided to swing by our trusted mechanic for one last ditch effort to find the part and do the programming that the dealer couldn't or wouldn't do. As I stood there defeated and frustrated in front of this mechanic, he was able to get the part and had the software to do the programming.

Although it would take a couple of weeks to get the part in, and it would still be very expensive to fix, it was not as expensive as a new car. So, we took the leap. We didn't know if fixing the TCM unit would ultimately fix *all* the problems, but everything we read and every test that was run pointed to a bad TCM unit.

Every symptom was pointing to this part of the electrical system of the car that was creating all of these physical breakdowns in the car that was leaving her broken down on the side of the road. So, we waited for the part to arrive and the appointment for the repair and programming. We had it installed by someone who knew what they were doing.

Guess what? It fixed everything! All of the damage was fixed. The shifting, the stalling, the poor gas mileage, the shutter and shakes, the power steering, the stereo, everything. All of these symptoms were because the electrical system was not able to send the correct information it needed. The battery, even though it was only a few months old, did need to be replaced because the draining of the electrical system compromised one of its cells.

We asked the question of why this TCM unit had gone bad because it's not a common problem. We found two reasons that the TCM unit goes bad. One reason being water damage, such as a flood. Obviously, water and electricity don't mix, but we knew this car had never experienced a flood.

Second reason was vibration.

Hmm, could it possibly have been the damage from a year earlier when the car had been driven at high rates of speed with a lot of vibration? We thought we had fixed all of the damage that had been done by that experience. But in fact, the TCM had been vibrated loose so that it wasn't having a good connection.

The first thing that went was the radio. But who would have ever connected that to the transmission? Over the year, it became worse and compounded until it shut the car down and ultimately had to be replaced.

Can you see how this story relates to you and your energy system? You may not know where a symptom comes from, especially if you can't see it.

If you have a dent in the fender, you can see it and repair it. In fact, the tires were the first indication of what happened to the car initially and we had replaced and repaired them because it was very physical and we could see the damage. Much like a knee or a shoulder injury, you know where the damage is so you can heal it.

What about the underlying damage in your energetic system that remains? Maybe it's even more insidious and you've had a loss or grief or an experience that hits your energetic system, but you don't recognize the impact of it because it's not physical. It's not visible or it's minimal. You keep on living and using your body the way you need to and the way you want to, just like she did with the car.

As the effects of the energetic disruption compound, it becomes impossible to ignore. It also becomes harder to recognize the underlying cause.

I had heard of this correlation of energy breakdowns being researched in breast cancer and thought it was fascinating. In fact, I had several friends diagnosed with breast cancer and each of them had experienced an extreme heartache with the death of a spouse or a child or a parent within the past 18 months.

Do not mistake my observation to say that you will get breast cancer from a death of a family member. My observation and examples are just to help you see the physical manifestation of a disruption in your energy systems. Likewise, the purpose of this system introduction is not to teach you how to repair it, but rather recognize it.

You can't change something you're not aware of. At this point, it's about learning to recognize what it feels like when your energy is hit, leaking, blocked, or just off. It's learning to not just fix the physical or superficial symptoms that are obvious, but to consider how it's landing or stemming from an energetic interference. Sometimes you can do your own energetic repair, and sometimes you may need to take it to an expert that can accurately identify and has the tools to fix the damage.

In the application section of this text, I will share energy hygiene and practical tools that you can use to keep your energy system running optimally. But as I mentioned, this metaphor is just about awareness. It's about recognizing that your physical body is an outward manifestation of what's happening in your energy body.

Some is obvious and familiar. Some is elusive and unfamiliar and maybe even woo woo.

System 2: Fuel

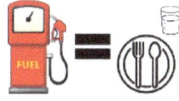

The second system in the framework to become the expert in your body is far more obvious and familiar to you, fuel. However, I'll preface with just because it's obvious and familiar does not mean that you have a healthy understanding of this system.

Why would you? The information that's fed to you, to all of us, in the Standard American Diet (SAD), is founded on old science, enormous marketing and lobby efforts from the food industry, and cultural norms and beliefs.

Do you feel like you're constantly being told different facts and studies about what is or isn't healthy to eat? Fat is bad. No, some fat is good. Fructose is bad. Wait, fructose is the natural sugar in fruit, and I thought fruit was good. Drink milk for strong bones. No, dairy causes cancer. You need to increase your protein to build muscle. Eat more meat. Hold on, meat causes heart disease.

To add insult to injury, you get drug into the dogma of certain diet programs and the vilification of their non approved foods. It's the all or nothing approach that gets results for the short term, but isn't sustainable, so you rebound back with a vengeance, right back to SAD. I'm thinking of diet camps like Atkins, vegan, keto, paleo, raw, carnivore.

Yes, it is true that more and more is being understood about the nutrients of certain foods and therefore the benefit to the body. Yes, it is true that more and more is being understood about the way the body interacts with and uses the food you eat. So, as I go into this system, I ask that you empty your cup.

Remember Lesson 5 from *8 Lessons Lupus Taught Me* and be open to learning how it applies to you, as you become the expert in your body. I ask for permission to remind you of things you may already know, as well as things that may be new to you, or challenge your beliefs.

How do you know your beliefs? Look at what you're eating, or not eating, and you'll get a glimpse of your beliefs about food. I also recognize that almost no one eats for nutrition.

As a speech language pathologist, I work with swallowing and feeding disorders. It is my job to recommend a feeding tube when an individual is unable to eat safely, and also my job to wean them off of tube feedings as they progress through therapy to help them use their muscles and automatic reflexes to protect their airway and swallow safely.

I also work with children who have sensory issues with feeding that result in overstimulation with avoidance, tantrums, or crying at even the proximity of a food in line of sight or smell. The taste and texture of certain foods may result in gagging and even vomiting. Systematically engaging them with positive experiences in controlled environments to retrain the nervous system to not overreact and to tolerate a wide variety of foods is my job.

These are extreme examples of how nutrition becomes the focus of eating, because without adequate nutrition the body breaks down and becomes malnourished, a literal diagnosis of failure to thrive. A body that is in a malnourished state cannot create healthy cells, which results in stunted growth, atrophy, and progression of disease processes.

Then there's another group, a more common group of us that eat for pleasure and comfort. This was the group I belonged to growing up, and still probably do to some degree.

Food was central to all family and social gatherings. More food equated to more safety. More food equated to more love. More food equated to more acceptance. Food was a way to serve and show compassion. Food was a way to share. Food was a delicious pleasure to be experienced and celebrated.

Finally, there's the group that I now belong to, and I'm going to hopefully convince you of the benefits to join me. This is the food as medicine group. This is where we celebrate and appreciate food, not just for the delicious pleasure and routine consumption, but also for the healing benefits.

Food is more than macros or calories. It's not an ethical dilemma of good versus bad. Food is a complex matrix of synergistic actions that supports your body in either cell growth, repair, and detoxification, or cell atrophy, mutation, and toxicity.

So it should be easy to know which foods are supportive and which are not, right? Well, yes, and in the grand scheme of food, that's where you get the banners of health food versus junk food. If I gave you a list of 20 foods, you would be able to categorize them accordingly. Remember though, that I am taking you to a new level of understanding, a level beyond what is good or bad, to a level of food as medicine.

This means that how a certain food interacts with your individual chemistry is important for you to recognize and manipulate in your lifestyle to heal your disease. You can't change something you're not aware of. So, you begin to categorize foods not just by their macros, protein, fat, carbohydrates, or calories, but by their complex matrix properties such as phytonutrients, polyphenols, antioxidants, anti-inflammatory, prebiotic, probiotic, etc.

As you understand your disease process, you begin to understand what types of food will support healthy repair and detoxification. For example, I am a self-proclaimed antioxidant junkie because the autoimmune disease of rheumatoid arthritis becomes extremely painful in my joints when I eat inflammatory foods.

I have spent time learning what foods are high in antioxidants and make sure that I eat them every day in every way so that the free radicals from oxidative stress I generate just by living every day can be hauled out of my body. I've also learned that my immune system is best supported when I eat plenty of pre and probiotic foods.

Initially, I resisted many of the fermented foods because they tasted awful. As my diet became more whole foods, produce diverse, and seasonal, my tastes changed and I now love them.

I later learned the reason for this phenomenon is that the microbiota in the gut are actually giving you the cravings for the foods you eat or resistance to the foods you won't eat. As the gut flora become healthier and more balanced, the cravings disappear.

Fuel in our human body is food and water, just like gas fuels a vehicle. However, the use and longevity of your living vehicle are far longer than your average car. Understanding the fuel you choose is important to maximize performance and longevity.

For example, for the failure to thrive vehicles, it's imperative to get the gas in to keep the car running. Consideration for macros, calories, and hydration is critical to ensure that there is continued safe nutrition to get through the disease crisis of this part of the journey. However, with the SAD vehicles, you'll find lines at the pump for the most convenient and economical gas.

Not a big deal unless you're driving a luxury or sports car that was made for premium. You know you can't put diesel in your car, so you don't choose the green nozzle, but you didn't realize that your car was engineered for premium. It can be a hassle to find the right octane level, and have you seen how expensive it is?

Filling up occasionally with regular gas doesn't seem to make a difference in how your car runs, so you don't worry about it. Until you end up broken down on the side of the road and the mechanic finds that the fuel you used compromised your engine. That is such a bummer.

Finally, the Food as Medicine vehicles are aware that they require premium gasoline to run optimally. You might even find them choosing a specific brand or using additives to clean the fuel line to enhance performance. This group understands their vehicle, journey, and driving conditions and adjust the fuel. Much like the pit crew of a racing team. Make no mistake about it, the type and quality of fuel matters, not just the quantity.

Sometimes it is obvious and results in an immediate breakdown, such as a night of too much alcohol or a food coma after a large meal. Most often, it is a slower process of poor quality over time that leads to poor performance and ultimately a breakdown such as autoimmune disease. The fantastic news is that fuel is the one thing that you can change with the least amount of effort and get the greatest amount of health.

With a little bit of education and evaluation, you can determine what the best food for you is and begin to make choices to pull up to a different pump. In time, you can have the skill and expertise of the pit crew to keep your vehicle in top performance condition, regardless of the journey.

That, my friend, is what we call thriving.

System 3: Maintenance

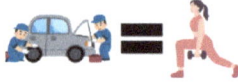

What maintenance equates to for the human body is self-care and movement because that is how we keep our systems in tip top shape. It's less intense or focused than nutrition because it's more routine and honestly easier to make excuses or let it go. Similar to our routine maintenance in comparison to our daily gasoline.

If you think about your car, you do routine maintenance every day. Your maintenance schedule is different based on the make, model, or age of your car. You wash it, you take out the trash, and you drive it within the parameters it was designed for. Hopefully.

If it's an older model, you may need to replace some hoses or have some systems flushed to maximize performance. If you're getting ready for a road trip, you might top off all your fluid levels, have your tires rotated and checked, and get new windshield wipers before you set out on your journey.

Similarly, we have to take care of our physical body the same way we take care of our car. It requires routine cleaning, inside and out, daily maintenance, and scheduled maintenance.

Routine cleaning includes not only your physical cleaning, but also your energetic cleaning. Remember System 1?

Moving your body is important just like it is for the car. I don't know if you've ever had a situation where your vehicle has had to be stored for a long period of time, but it's not good for it. It drains the battery, the fluids settle and can create problems in the engine, and the hoses and seals can dry and crack.

Interestingly, the same is true for your body. Have you ever noticed how sitting around scrolling or watching TV drains your energy and you aren't motivated to get up and go to the gym?

For me, extended sitting gives me the stiffies. That's what I call it when I try to get up, especially quickly, and my body reminds me that my joints have settled and I need to move a little bit before I can get my actual movement in gear.

It's amazing to me how quickly atrophy sets in when you're down sick or out of your routine and not regularly moving your body the way it was designed to be used; like walking, bending, lifting, squatting, throwing, catching, jogging, etc.

Hoorah! We are designed to be active beings. Think of a physical activity that you did in your youth but you haven't done since. Could you get up and do it right now? Would it look the same as it did when you used to do it?

I used to be on the dance team in high school, but other than dancing in my kitchen or with my husband on rare occasions, I haven't done a routine in decades.

When my youngest daughter was in high school a few years ago, I was asked to participate in a tradition for her dance team as a member of the parent team. Wow, I didn't remember the choreography the way I used to! I was far more self-conscious and nervous than I used to be. Some of the other parents were still dancers who own and operate dance studios. They were still able to remember the choreography and have no problem being the star of the show.

I use this as an example because I love to dance, but because I haven't done that type of dance in ages, it was awkward and challenging. I still have the flexibility to do the splits after a little warmup because I've used my body in similar ways with yoga staying limber and strong. But because I haven't used all of my body in that physical activity, it took me some time to be able to master it to a performance level.

My system needed to be flushed and restarted because it had been out of commission for too long.

You know what routine maintenance looks like for your car, and you know that sometimes it gets put off or moved down the priority list. How about your routine maintenance? What is known as self-care.

I observe two groups of people when I speak of self-care. One that is rampant in the autoimmune community is the Shero. Too busy taking care of everyone else to have time, money, or energy to take care of yourself. Maybe there's even an underlying belief that your significant other, kids, job, church, education, (fill in your blank) is more important than taking care of you.

You are a selfless person that puts everyone else and their needs before yours. I talk about this indirectly in lesson 4 Health is #1 in the book *8 Lessons Lupus Taught Me: From Surviving to Thriving with Autoimmune Diseases*. It's the analogy of the airline safety lesson, where you're told to put on your own oxygen mask before you help the dependents traveling with you.

The reality is if you don't do your own self-care, and do it first, you will not be able to continue to be that Shero that you are.

The other group I call Vanity Fair. Worried about keeping up appearances and having a perfect image, but it's all a facade. Comparing yourself to everyone else, you don't go to the gym because it's not the right gym. You don't want anyone else to see you without makeup because you feel like you look ugly. You don't have the right clothes to exercise. You fill in the excuse.

This group has had insult added to the injury with social media and the comparison trap of someone else's edited life becoming the standard of comparison for your real unedited life.

This group is hiding from life because they feel like they can't measure up. You can't get out of the garage. I certainly have found myself in both of these groups at different times in my life. It's important that you recognize them both as beliefs that are sabotaging your critical maintenance schedule and will no doubt land you in the shop.

What is your service record? What do your excuses tell you about your beliefs? Where are your priorities for self-care?

To bring it back to the vehicle metaphor, do you clean the trash out every day? Do you stop at the car wash occasionally and get the cheapest wash because you can't stand it anymore or do you schedule regularly for the full detail?

Are you rotating your tires regularly so that they are lasting longer? Or are you waiting until the tread has uneven wear and the result is a blowout?

How are you driving? Are you driving Mach 10 with your hair on fire and constantly road raging against the idiots around you? Are you riding your brakes and burning them out?

Do you use your car as a dining room and allow others to schlep their mud in and out leaving a mess for you to clean up?

What grade of oil and gasoline are you using and is it what is recommended for your specific car? Every vehicle comes with an owner's manual that gives you the recommended maintenance schedule and the grade of oil and type of gasoline to use. The same is true for us as people.

It doesn't matter what reason you have for not maintaining the car. There will be consequences of poor performance, expensive repairs, and eventually an early retirement to the junkyard or crushing machine. Learning what your ideal self-care routine and schedule is, and doing it consistently is critical to optimal performance, or what I call thriving.

It's important to put away the limiting beliefs that you can't do self-care, or you don't deserve self-care. Because, if you don't, you will break down. Living WOW has recommended daily, monthly, and seasonal self-care schedules and routines that give you the structure to maximize your performance. You learn what your ideal self-care routine and schedule is by making it a priority.

As you implement it regularly, you realize you have more quality time to spend with those you love because you have more energy. You have more money because you aren't spending it on co-pays, deductibles, and medications. An ounce of prevention is yet again, better than a pound of cure. Priceless!

System 4: Oil

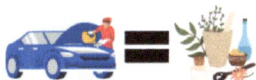

System four, oil, relates to supplements in the human body. This is a system that's kind of a subsystem because it's related to your fuel, but it's not the same as your fuel. You have to have oil to keep your engine working properly.

It's also part of maintenance because you have to change it routinely. Which oil you use depends on your vehicle, much like your fuel and other required maintenance.

Systems 2 fuel, 3 maintenance, and 4 oil, all have an interconnectedness, but I break them out because they each have a different purpose, schedule, and focus. Oil is what I refer to as supplements. It supports the fuel system, and it helps the engine to work optimally. Good oil and clean oil really help your system run well.

If your oil has leaked out and you keep driving it, your engine has the potential to burn up. That is the analogy I use for supplements. Can you run without supplements? Yes, for a time, but you can't have optimal performance.

Not all oil is created equal. Not all supplements are created equal.

Supplementation is important because our food does not provide all of the nutrients that our bodies need. We have greater demands to offload toxins because there are more toxins in our modern society than there ever have been. Additionally, because of growing and marketing conditions, many foods are nutrient deficient so it takes a greater amount to get those necessary nutrients.

Some of the nutrients are just lacking as your life season changes. For teens versus adults versus a senior, the same body metabolizes differently and absorbs nutrients differently. Therefore, you need more of certain things at different times of your life. Additionally, if you're sick, you are going to benefit from supplementation.

It's not meant to be something that you do all the time like fuel. That's where understanding what you need and when you need it to build up your system is important. The reason that over the counter, run of the mill, traditional multivitamins (think Flintstones or Centrum) don't work is that the body doesn't absorb them.

Is it better than nothing? Yes. Is it optimal? No. Of course, with Living WOW you want everything to be optimal because you want to heal systems that are broken down, maintain them, and thrive, not just survive.

When you're looking at supplementation, you want to make sure you're addressing bioavailability. Can that supplement get into your system and do what it's designed to do?

The problem is that so often when we take 15 vitamins that we know are good for us and isolate them, it fractionates them. I talked about the importance of the whole food matrix back in System 2 Fuel. Food has thousands of nutrients in a single apple, or in a single broccoli, or in a single leaf of spinach.

And they're all different. Many are the same. But many of them we don't even know. Those foods offer different benefits, and when they're eaten as a whole food, it works like magic in your body. Not only is it bioavailable, but your body uses the whole food matrix to support it exactly where you need it.

You don't have to guess what nutrient you need to support your brain, or your heart, or your liver. The whole food matrix is like magic in that it knows and supports what you need, not just what is recommended.

Science has tried to recreate that benefit by extracting the most recognized vitamins and minerals like vitamin C, vitamin A, vitamin E, calcium, magnesium, or beta carotene, and putting them in the optimal recommended daily allowance into a multivitamin.

It's so convenient. You can take them and think you have your bases covered. The problem is that isolated, fractionated, or synthetic vitamin, mineral, or supplement is not as valuable to your body as a whole food based or naturally produced supplement. So always research the source of your supplement.

Because the supplement industry is loosely monitored, fillers and unlisted ingredients can actually do harm. You may remember the GNC sting that occurred a few years back when products were taken off the shelf, independently tested, and found to have illegal and unlisted ingredients in some of the supplements sold.

Now, let's not throw the baby out with the bathwater and assume that all supplements are unnecessary or harmful. Remember, your body is not getting optimal nutrition with food alone. This is true no matter what diet you're eating. This lesson really hit home to me and was the initial catalyst of my health transformation that I wrote about in *8 Lessons Lupus Taught Me: From Surviving to Thriving with Autoimmune Diseases*.

To set the stage, I was going into my 40th birthday overweight, exhausted, with chronic pain from rheumatoid arthritis that I had been living with for 15 years. I knew that I needed to lose weight, but with every diet I would end up losing 10 pounds and gaining 20 back. That's how I got to be 80 pounds overweight to begin with.

I watched a presentation at a Toastmasters group about Juice Plus+® and thought it was an incredible idea, but didn't really think I needed it and dismissed it. A couple of weeks later, I heard another presentation at a Women and Children's Networking group about Juice Plus+® Children's Health Study. This time, I couldn't ignore it.

I had been worried about my daughter's nutrition and realized that maybe this would help, and it certainly couldn't hurt. I signed us up for this study, hoping to see her food cravings change, but not really having any other expectations.

Fast forward about six weeks later and I'm sitting at my desk finishing up a long day of charting and my hands didn't hurt. I couldn't remember the last time my hands didn't hurt so it really got my attention.

What was in those capsules of produce that no medication, therapy, doctor, or supplement had? This is when I ran headlong into nutritional healing. It was also when I signed up my husband and other kids to eat Juice Plus+® and became a representative.

Since that day in May 2009, I've been advocating for whole food supplementation because it literally changed my life. I couldn't believe that despite working in health care for 15 years, including doing feeding and swallowing therapies, that I didn't know about this product. I didn't realize that despite eating a "good diet" and taking a regimen of 10 supplements daily, my pain would be eliminated through whole food capsules.

Fifteen years later, I continue to eat Juice Plus+® and recommend it with confidence because it is my foundational supplement. Because it is food, it gets into the body and works the same synergistic magic that happens when you eat the whole food in its raw form. The difference is that I'm able to get the quantity, quality, and diversity for my body that I'm not able to get with my meals only.

I am confident about the bioavailability, not only because of my own experience, but also the reputation as a highly researched product at prestigious universities around the world, proving that it not only gets into the body, but it supports the systems.

It was exciting to learn and understand why the produce in the capsules took away my pain and have it also validated by research. They now have even more research including five studies on inflammation and 18 on bioavailability. Those two, inflammation and bioavailability, are super important to me.

Remember the hesitancy I mentioned you should have about supplements because of what's in them, unlisted ingredients, or maybe what's not, like fillers?

I also recommend Juice Plus+® confidently to family, friends, and you because of the third-party testing and certifications on all of their products. I have been to the packaging facility in California and witnessed firsthand the level of quality control that goes into the products. As a Juice Plus+® partner, I see the care and ethics that go into the supplement.

In fact, because it is a whole food product, it actually falls under the food category and is not allowed to have a supplement label because it only contains food so it has a nutrition label. I still prefer to refer to it as a supplement because it does not replace my food (think fuel). It supplements it (think oil).

Just like with your food, I recommend you turn it over and read the ingredient list, not just the label. When I'm looking for an additional supplement like vitamin D3, for example, I'm careful to research the company that distributes it, making sure they're reputable and not on the sting list, and then do my own due diligence reading the ingredients.

I am continually amazed by fillers and sugars added to supplements. They're just not necessary and may be harmful. I no longer have a 10 vitamin daily regimen, but I absolutely do recommend supplementation. If you could have optimal performance with diet alone, you would not see so many of the diseases that are rampant in our world today.

You need supplements. Listen to your body and understand how age, activity level, and even where you live can factor into what additional support your body would benefit from. I now eat Juice Plus+® as my daily foundation supplements that includes the veg, fruits, berries, and omega blends, and add in other nutrients as I need them like D3, magnesium, zinc, etc. for shorter durations.

Bringing it back to the car analogy, to understand how you are the expert in your body for Living WOW, remember supplements are like oil. Quality and quantity matter with oil. Similar to fuel, but still different and no less important to the overall performance of your car.

If you are running on sludgy oil or your oil level is too low, you are absolutely looking at significant damage to your car. If left unchecked long enough, your car will eventually break down. On the flip side, routine oil changes will give you optimal performance and extend the miles your car will take you.

That's what I call thriving.

System 5: The Driver

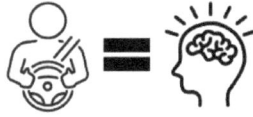

Who is driving your vehicle? Well, your mind, of course. Your mind is an interesting character because it's made up of both a physical organ, your brain, and an energetic intelligence that is eternal.

I think of the mind as the bridge that connects the physical body and the energetic spiritual body so that the two realms cross over and communicate in their respective roles.

Now, before you check out, because I'm getting too woo woo on you, consider opening your mind to the concepts, capabilities, and limitations of your mind as the driver of your car in the 8 systems framework.

When I refer to mind, I am referring to both the physical characteristics of the brain, the way the chemicals and neurons send and receive signals in the physical space in your brain, as well as the energetic, spiritual, intelligence characteristics of the mind. The conscious and subconscious thought processes.

Let's start with the physical brain because it's the most easily recognized and understood. The brain literally tells you how to drive the car. The physical characteristics of starting the car, shifting gears, understanding and using safety features like seat belts and turn signals, and checking your mirrors for other vehicles are completed by the brain as it tells your arms, legs, and head how to perform the physical actions necessary.

Your mind takes over as it looks over the environment around you, searching for threats to getting to your destination. Your mind recognizes the light turning from yellow to red and makes a decision of whether you should stop or go, depending on the risk assessment of how much time and traffic you have to stop suddenly or speed up to make the light.

Maybe you've been sitting at a red light with no other cars in sight and your mind says, "Just go. There's no reason to sit here and wait for it to turn green." There is no threat. Similarly, your mind tells your brain when the conditions are dangerous to be alert. Send more adrenaline to keep the senses and reflexes sharp because you may have an accident and not get to your destination.

This is the activation of the sympathetic nervous system, which you likely recognize as the fight, flight, or freeze response. Everything the mind does is for the purpose of getting you to your destination. Your mind is constantly analyzing and processing the conditions, threats, opportunities, and vehicle function.

Your mind follows the directions it's told, whether it be from the signs, other drivers, or the navigation system. It functions similarly to a computer processing data to provide a particular outcome.

What happens when you drive distracted? Sometimes nothing. Have you ever been driving and you suddenly realize that you don't remember driving the last mile or two of your journey? Your mind checked out and went on autopilot, with your brain running the physical aspects with muscle memory, while your mind processed something else it recognized as more important or interesting than your boring drive that you've driven a million times.

Until the truck in front of you hits its brakes. Thank goodness it was huge so you saw it and had time to hit your brakes. Phew, that was a close call. Wait, everyone is hitting their brakes! Four lanes of traffic are stopped. What's going on? Suddenly, the mind is searching for threats and explanations. After a mile of creeping along, watching the time because now you're running late, you finally see flashing emergency lights and eventually drive by the demolished vehicles from a high speed multi car accident and send up a prayer for those involved, hoping that they survived.

In the past five miles of your journey, the driver has gone from autopilot, to threat detection and response, to threat detection and worry, to threat recognition and response. How your driver processes and responds to those environmental triggers is dependent upon your age, experience, beliefs, and vehicle.

Can you see how this analogy plays out in your larger journey of life? It's important to understand the role of the mind and the impact of the information you feed it. Running in a constant state of stress and overstimulation will result, at best, in a breakdown, and at worst, devastating accident.

You've heard the adage "garbage in, garbage out". Often used in reference to junk food and poor health. What about the habits, distractions, and information you're putting into your mind? What are you reading? What are you listening to? What are you looking at? Who are you spending time with? What are you learning? Do you know where you're going? Are you consuming junk thoughts or healthy thoughts?

Although there definitely is a cumulative effect with junk food, by and large I believe it to be less destructive than junk thoughts. The body is built to filter and release toxins, so generally the junk food is out of your system within a couple of days. Not true with the mind, which is built to retain every thought you have ever had and file it away in case you may need it for reference to survive one day.

In fact, the mind latches onto the most threatening thoughts and puts them on a loop so that you have less of a chance of experiencing that same threat again.

Don't believe me? Are you perseverating on the compliment a coworker gave you today or the criticism someone else had of you yesterday? Are you glancing into the mirror as you wash your hands, thinking how beautiful you look or noticing that your hair is flat?

Do you recognize how all of your organs are functioning perfectly and automatically or the ache in your back today? Are you afraid because of news reports of crime and calamities or do you realize that you're safe and that most people are good and helpful?

It's not because you're a negative Nellie. You're wired for survival, and as such, your mind is wired with a negativity bias. A protection mechanism meant to keep you safe. However, in the modern world, much like bodies are overtaxed with toxins, the mind is overtaxed with stimulation and information.

Diligence to filter what you allow in your mind dictates what the mind will loop. Your mind will always gravitate to the negative threat, so consciously filling the mind with active and intentional stimulation and information is the best way to hack the negativity bias.

Similar to the healthy strategy of choosing 'this, not that' when eliminating junk food. You can do the same thing with junk thoughts.

Choose intentional rather than automatic. An example may be to learn a new skill rather than scroll social media. The mind is then active in learning and not picking up on derogatory posts or snide memes.

Engage a new intention filter and go back to the habits, distractions, and information you are allowing into your mind.

What are you reading? What are you listening to? What are you looking at? Who are you spending time with? What are you learning? Where are you going? Awareness makes all the difference in the world.

Awareness of junk thoughts is much more difficult, and the lack of awareness is much more insidious. Your body cannot function optimally and thrive if the driver isn't healthy.

Like a computer released to the wild internet frontier with no firewalls, antivirus software, malware protection, or security feature, it's only a matter of time until corruption takes hold and shuts it down. However, fortified with the right protection, you can identify risks and routinely scan for threats in a healthy way, being proactive rather than reactive.

Coming back to the driver analogy, it's important to recognize that the driver has a distinct role separate from the vehicle, and without the driver, the car is useless. With that said, the driver is limited to only taking in information and processing it.

Likewise, the driver has a negativity bias programmed to keep you safe and get you to the destination, but in the modern world can completely shut you down with overstimulation and system failure.

By understanding the role and tendencies of the driver, you can support optimal processing and operation. A strong and focused driver is a critical part of your journey to thriving.

System 6: Navigation

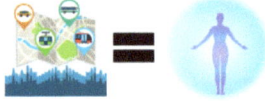

I spoke briefly of the navigation system during the introduction of the driver of System 5. Remember that the driver does what it's told with the purpose of getting you to your destination safely. But how do you know where to go? System 6, Navigation! Your navigation system.

You will see navigation helps all along the journey. This may be in the form of signs, maps, or even other drivers giving you information that was useful to them.

What is unique and personal to you, however, is your personal navigation system. Your navigation system is beyond high tech. Your navigation system knows not only where you are going, but also all of the side roads, detours, and reroutes that you may need to encounter on your journey.

It is critical that the driver tunes into the personal navigation system because it can be easily drowned out by the noise of the journey and the driving conditions. Every time I think of this system, I reflect back to when I first learned to trust my navigation system.

I was on a quick weekend trip to watch my oldest daughter play tennis in a community six hours from our home. I was somewhat familiar with the route, but had not driven the road before. It was spring, so I packed accordingly for myself and my other two children, ages infant and 11 years. We were ready for a fun weekend getaway. We left after my son got out of school, but most of the drive would still be in the dark.

I had my reliable Road Atlas with me because I wasn't completely sure of the route details, and I always made sure I had it with me for road trips. My husband had bought a Garmin GPS and thought it would be a great opportunity to use it.

We had played with it a little around town with lots of rerouting and buffering and funny pronunciations of some local roads. This new technology was mostly entertainment at that point, but a road trip was the perfect opportunity to give it a go. I set my hotel address as the destination in my GPS, kissed my husband goodbye, buckled up the kids, and off we went. Everything went as planned until we were about two hours away from home.

Darkness had set in, and as we started into the mountain pass, we were greeted by an unexpected snowfall. Initially, I talked to the kids about the snow and how it was not in the forecast. It was so dark that we couldn't see the beauty of it and the kids fell asleep. I had not prepared for snow. I had only considered the weather at home and the weather for the tennis tournament.

What I thought was a spring flurry became a whiteout. Zero visibility. On a mountain road that I was unfamiliar with, I was beginning to get nervous. If we slid off the road, we were not prepared for these conditions. If I pulled off the road, it would be just as dangerous, potentially causing an accident because there was no shoulder and no visibility.

I then began to realize that not only did I have zero visibility, but the signs were completely covered with snow. They offered me no anchor as to where I was, how much farther I had to go to get to civilization, or what kind of help may be ahead. After what felt like an eternity, I heard a somewhat familiar voice tell me to turn left in 10 miles.

That was when I realized that my GPS was still navigating and could see through the storm when I could not. It had been quiet for hours because there was nothing to tell me as we navigated over the pass with no turns or stops required. I started watching the map on my GPS to give me information about where I was on my journey, when I would be able to stop and get gas, and what my ETA was.

Despite being on a mountain pass with no cell phone coverage, the GPS navigation system worked. My usual navigation devices were useless on this trip because I couldn't see the road signs and I couldn't pull over to read a map in the dark in the middle of a blizzard. I didn't have anyone with me that was familiar with the road any more than I was.

I quickly learned to rely on and trust the GPS navigation system. We made it to our destination late in the night, but safe and sound. The next day, as we basked in the sun at the tennis tournament, there was no sign of the tenuous journey through the blinding snow we had endured the night before. The lesson had been learned, and my opinion of this silly technology had been elevated.

In applying this metaphor to our journey of life and the Living WOW system's framework, you may have realized that the navigation system is your spirit. Your nonphysical being is an eternal intelligence and interacts with God and other spirit beings. Not much is really known about the spiritual being because it's not seen and therefore cannot be studied and understood as our physical bodies can.

As such, there are many beliefs, customs, and religions that attempt to define and teach about the spirit. My purpose is not to comment on any beliefs, customs, or religions. Of course, I do recognize my bias as a believer in God, Jesus Christ, and the Holy Spirit, and how I relate to my personal spirit and the spiritual realm.

I believe that my spirit is a divine and eternal intelligence, and as such has a connection to the divine realm and all that is in it. I believe that God is the Supreme Creator of all. I have a purpose, as all creation does. God is aware of my purpose, my destination, and my journey. We have been given general guides for our destination and journey with scriptures, prophets, teachers, and parents.

But your spirit is the only one that knows the details of your journey in real time. That's why I refer to it as a guide. As your "voice of truth". You may refer to it as your instinct or gut feeling. Every single one of us has a spirit body, but how you recognize and interact with it is unique to you.

I will often interchange energy and spirit because they exist in the same realm. But to me, energy is the bigger interaction within the universe and spirit is my personal connection to my Creator. They very much interact like my mind and body physically interact, but they have distinct designations within the system's framework.

To conceptualize it, the energy body is much like the physical body in structure and function, while the spirit is much like the mind in structure and function. The spirit oversees and navigates the journey, while the mind processes the information and drives the vehicle.

The problem is that you may have never heard your navigation system, and certainly never learned to trust it. The noise of the driving conditions or the overwhelming information and distractions that the driver keeps fixating on is all you can hear.

Maybe it's just unfamiliar technology and seems unnecessary. Maybe it's been quiet for so long you forgot it's still there. I would encourage you to take it for a test drive.

The simplest way I know is what I call prayer. If you don't pray, just find a quiet space and ponder or meditate on a question you have about your journey. The key is to get quiet and eliminate distractions so that you can tune in and hear your voice of truth. You don't have to have a certain format or routine or place or time.

The cool thing about your spirit is that, just like your body, it's unique to you. As you begin to listen, you will recognize what your voice of truth sounds like. It is never self-deprecating, defeating, or hostile. Those are the lies that your mind has picked up from living SAD. Learning to quiet the mind and listen to the spirit is the key to successful navigation on your journey to living your best life.

This is the most misunderstood and underrated system in the framework. If you can learn to listen to your spirit and trust that it is connected to the Creator's Spirit, you will find the peace and healing that is elusive in the world.

Bringing it back to the metaphor, know that your spirit is your internal, individually programmed navigation system that is prepared for your journey. You can always trust it, because the system never fails, even when the external navigation guides are not available or give you mixed messages. Know that your navigation system is always connected and running, even when you don't hear it above the noise of the road.

System 7:
The Indicator Lights

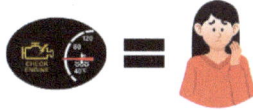

Your body is telling you what it needs. Are you listening? Are you too busy to hear it? Do you know the language of your body? Are you experiencing deep fatigue? Irritable bowels? Diarrhea? Bloating? Constipation? Headaches? Brain fog? Rashes? Do you have pain? Where at and what kind?

Some symptoms may appear universal, but actually can be specific and telling. When you begin to understand what is happening in your body, it speaks the answers that can help lead you to the underlying trigger.

A personal example for me is an infection that I'm prone to get on my face and my nose. That infection is related to lupus. I know what is happening with my immune system when this infection blossoms.

I have learned that I can look back and see the trigger event, usually three to five days prior. It is usually an emotional event that triggered a stress response in my body. Then that stress response cascades in my body, shutting down my immune response, which sets the environment for the opportunistic infection to kick into hyperdrive as it rebounds and begins attacking its system of choice, which for me is usually the lungs, the brain, or the skin. Having this infection recur year after year, I've learned what it means and how to get in front of it.

I also have specific symptoms of rheumatoid arthritis. These are more related to my diet. When I eat foods that are inflammatory, such as sugar or processed foods, I then feel more stiffness, swelling, and pain.

I know that the emotional triggers that trigger my lupus flares are different than the dietary triggers that trigger my arthritis flares.

These are my personal examples of what I call the indicator lights because they are most familiar to me. I know you have your own indicator lights. This is also the reason that I say that I love my autoimmune diseases and I feel blessed to have them because my body will give me early warning signs.

Not everyone is so fortunate. But you are, if you learn to recognize and heed the warning.

Most inflammation, systemic inflammation, you don't feel. Oxidative stress, free radical damage, and inflammation throughout your body is unrecognized in our SAD lifestyle, perpetuated by high stress, high anxiety, increasing chaos, and low to no rest and recovery.

Because it is so common, it's become normalized to be sick and tired, so you push on. If your symptoms become intrusive enough, you may go to your doctor, who gives you medication to relieve the symptom. But without relieving the symptom entirely, you find yourself with a new set of symptoms from what is affectionately termed 'side effects'.

Going back to my first example of the infection, this pattern went back as far as 1999. It was 12 years before this was linked to lupus, and another 5 years before I learned the pattern. It took another 5 years before I learned how to get in front of it rather than respond to the impending flare.

Now I can look back and see the obvious pattern. But then I was living SAD with a high stress lifestyle, working in a high stress medical crisis environment, triggered by a series of emotional losses. There was no way my body was prepared for the incoming perceived threats coming at me. So I ran, completely unaware, and continued running in fight and flight until the infection took hold.

The doctor treated me for a staph infection with antibiotics, which then led to an overgrowth of yeast, which then required antifungals. A few weeks later, the infection would recur. New antibiotics, antivirals, antifungals, topical steroids, the list of prescriptions and the resulting side effects just kept growing.

The cycle continued for years across multiple doctors and specialists. It wasn't until a completely unrelated set of symptoms sent me to a new specialist and a biopsy for a completely different condition, which resulted in the diagnosis of systemic lupus erythematosus.

That's when I woke up, but I still didn't recognize or understand the indicator lights.

This is why I share my personal story. I lived this cycle for years doing what everyone told me to do and what everyone else was doing because I didn't understand the language of my body. I had never been taught that my body had the answer all along, if I would just take the time to learn and listen what it was trying to tell me.

Resist the urge to suppress your symptoms and, even more drastically, suppress your immune system. Because those are your indicator lights. Instead, track them.

Track your symptoms. They tell you which system to pay attention to. If it's your digestion, do a journal of your food. Grab the low hanging fruit first. The easiest things to change and the easiest things to see effects are when you change your diet.

If you switch from inflammatory foods, or foods that you may have a sensitivity to. Maybe it's just inflammatory foods, like processed foods, gluten, dairy, sugar, alcohol, caffeine, that are triggering. When you eliminate those journal and track, that's it.

You can start to learn what your inflammatory triggers are. What are you most sensitive to? What are your super foods that relieve your symptoms and make you feel amazing? This is what happened in my personal experience where I was able to completely eliminate my rheumatoid arthritis symptoms with my diet.

But then I had my diagnosis of oral lichen planus and lupus. When I looked back, I had experienced the symptoms of lupus for many years, but it had never been diagnosed. My nutrition had relieved my chronic fatigue, and I felt better than I had in my adult life, but I still had enough systemic damage going on that my indicator lights were going off.

I knew it wasn't my nutrition, because I was experiencing so much positive effect in my body.

I knew there still had to be something more. And that is when I started looking at lifestyle. What was happening with my energetic state? What was happening with my mood? I literally felt like I had bipolar disorder because I was so up and down.

Depression and anxiety that weren't my typical energetic and outgoing, fun-loving self. I was mean, I was irritable, and I was snappy. When I did a deep dive into my lifestyle, I realized the impact of the energetic body and emotion with the interaction of my work environment, my relationships, my belief systems, and how I navigated through all of those energies.

I started to understand the things I couldn't see and how they physically manifested in my body. As I learned more about the interplay within my body and my lifestyle choices, I began to recognize behaviors that would support a healthy immune response or catapult me into a systemic autoimmune response.

I would encourage you to take a look at your autoimmune disease and each symptom. Which system is your body attacking? Is it Crohn's disease or celiac disease, which is leading you to the gut, the digestive system? Are you dealing with Hashimoto's or Graves disease, which is leading you to the thyroid and the endocrine system?

Are you dealing with psoriasis or lichen planus, which is leading you to the skin and the integumentary system? Are you dealing with spondylitis or arthritis, which is leading you to the bones and joints of the musculoskeletal system? Are you dealing with multiple sclerosis or systemic lupus, which is leading you to the nervous system?

Learning a new language takes time, but your indicator lights are critical and worth the effort to figure them out. They are also always accurate. Even when you don't understand. Your body is innately designed to heal and your symptoms are telling you where your environment is preventing healing or causing the damage.

Ignoring the symptoms by masking or suppressing is similar to putting black tape over the dashboard of your car. You have no idea what is really going on in any system. As one system impacts another, it is only a matter of time until the car blows up or breaks down.

Just as the indicator lights on the dash of your car tell you where you need to begin looking for support and repair, your symptoms can tell you where to begin looking for needed support and repair.

Once you begin to recognize the symptom as an indicator light, you can begin to learn the language of your body. You can methodically begin to break it down and listen to your body rather than suppressing the symptoms or the immune response.

Your indicator lights can help you recognize the causes or triggers of your autoimmune response and help you heal rather than layering on coping mechanisms.

Awareness is valuable because if you can get to the cause, then you can start to tweak your lifestyle to determine what is contributing to your disease and ultimately thrive because of it rather than suffer and survive with it.

System 8:
Driving Conditions

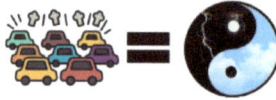

As we wrap up the 8 Systems Framework, it's worthwhile to point out that this final system is both external and internal. I include it in the 8 Systems Framework because it's impossible to separate yourself from or ignore the driving conditions completely.

Additionally, for the most part, you have very little, if any, control over the driving conditions. With that said, you must be aware of what they are and how they affect your vehicle and the journey so that you don't end up in an accident or breakdown due to unsafe or undesirable conditions. I've alluded to driving conditions in other examples throughout this series.

The first one I shared with you during System 1 when I shared the example of my teenage daughter and the transmission control unit, the TCM unit, that was the underlying cause of many malfunctions in the electrical system of her vehicle. The car had been driven at high speeds, drifting, burning the rubber off the tires, and creating an extreme vibration in the car.

We were aware of the damage done to the tires, brakes, and alignment, but not to the electrical system. This was an example of driving conditions that were outside of the car's capacity.

I also shared in System 6, the need for my reliance on the Garmin GPS system as I navigated through an unexpected spring snowstorm with my young children, completely unprepared for the conditions, both for the car and for the passengers.

I was focused on getting the little kids packed and ready for the six-hour road trip and planning on meeting up with my oldest daughter and her high school tennis team at the tournament. I had only checked the weather at home and at our destination for packing purposes. I had given no thought to the road other than the route as it was unfamiliar to me.

This was an example of driving conditions that were unavoidable at the time, but fortunately for me, I was more prepared than I realized.

Driving conditions in a vehicle are everything from traffic to weather, overdue maintenance, and fuel levels. You have little to no control over traffic and weather. Maintenance and fuel you have control over if you have the knowledge of what to do and when, and you plan accordingly.

How you respond to these conditions is the result of your beliefs and experience. Do you avoid heavy traffic, night driving or inclement weather or do you just keep on trucking? Do you top off your tank frequently or run on empty? Do you rotate your tires every 3, 000 miles or when they have to be replaced? Do you run on premium gas and oil, or get by with the cheapest option to keep you on the road?

The metaphor of the driving conditions directly ties to the lifestyle choices we make and the SAD culture we live in. The social norms, cultural beliefs, political and economic conditions are largely outside of our control, much like weather and traffic.

Learning how to optimize your body's health and performance with lifestyle choices is completely within your control, if you have the knowledge of what to do and when, and then you plan accordingly.

Like the driving conditions, the circumstances around us are continually changing. Some you may be able to plan for and some will come out of nowhere, completely derailing your journey.

Living WOW was created as a framework for lifestyle awareness, education, and resources to optimize health and vitality. Recognizing that you live in a SAD environment, much of what you have no control over. You do have complete control over how you respond and prepare for the circumstances around you.

There may be times when you're blindsided with a diagnosis, but know that as you learn to listen and understand the language of your body and become the expert in your body, you will recognize how all 8 systems work individually, yet inextricably together. Maybe it's time to put the car in the shop for some overdue maintenance.

Now that you're more familiar with the 8 systems, you have a better understanding of which kind of mechanic you need. Maybe you need to learn more about the fuel and maintenance of your vehicle's make, model, and mileage.

Maybe you need a mechanic that can help you understand why your energetic system is down regulating and potentially affecting other systems.

Maybe you need a mechanic that can help the driver and the navigation system to better work together, to not just get you to the destination, but to recognize the joy in the journey.

Understanding these 8 systems is the first step to becoming the expert in your own body.

Let's dive into the next step as we move into application of learning to speak the language of your body's systems. In the following chapters, we will dive deeper into each system, connecting you with the tools, resources, and providers that can help you build your own WOW lifestyle thriving on your journey.

Application

Grab a piece of paper and write down these numbers. You're going to go over the 8 systems of the Living WOW framework and rate from zero to ten in your lifestyle today.

Resist the urge to give the "right" answer. There is no right answer, only your honest answer. You can't change something you're not aware of so let's use this as an opportunity to get honest and take inventory.

0 (zero) being you have either no awareness of it or it's something you really struggle with. You are surviving.

10 (ten) being you've mastered it. You totally understand and are intentional. You are thriving.

System 1~Energy

Do you have enough energy to be able to run full out? Do you have the energy to live the life you want to live? Are you aware of the energies around you and how they interact with your energy? Do you have an energy hygiene routine that keeps your systems clean and flowing?

On a scale of 0-10 where would you rate your awareness, understanding, and resources of your energy system? Zero being that you have little to no awareness, maybe even fear of energy work. Ten being that you are aware and able to recognize energy hits, blocks, leaks, or damage and the tools to move and heal them.

System 2~ Fuel

Are you intentional with the foods you eat and drink? Are you eating for the seasons? Are you eating on the run, grab and go?

What's in season where you live? That's the first place you can start. Do you have a farmer's market? Can you go see what the farmers are selling? Because if it's not at the farmer's market, it's not in season.

I will tell you, I live in a high desert of the United States in Idaho. I love pineapple, mango, avocados. I love oranges, grapefruit, and bananas. None of those are in season for me ever because I don't live in that climate.

You can tell out of region what is in season usually by the price at the grocery store. When the price goes on sale it is usually because it is in season, more available, and more fresh. When the price goes up it is usually out of season, less available, and less fresh.

So, the things that are in season for me, if I'm eating for the season locally is berries. All sorts of berries, lettuces, and greens are thriving right now. This summer it'll be peppers, tomatoes, eggplants, cucumbers, beans, peas, and all kinds of veg. That's what's in season where I live. Stone fruits including apricots, plums, and cherries are on right now with peaches and apples available at the end of summer.

This doesn't mean you don't eat foods that aren't from where you live. Because we live in a modern age where we're able to get those. And what a blessing and how cool that is, because my favorite foods are tropical! Rather, be aware and take those cues from nature.

How are you doing? Zero, you have no awareness, you just eat whatever's in front of you. It's usually frozen or it's a drive thru. Maybe it's coming from a box or a can so it has no season. Versus 10, you're eating for the seasons, you're eating locally, maybe you're even growing your own. You've got your food dialed in.

Don't forget your water. You're going to need to increase your water intake if it's summer, because summer you're sweating and evaporating more. Hydration is essential for your body to function properly. Water is how your body moves the nutrients and oxygen through your system and takes out the waste is through water.

Much like food, not all hydration is created equal. Good clean water is supreme over all other hydration much like whole foods is supreme over all processed foods.

You may find it boring or need some pick me up or calm you down from other beverages. Not a problem, just be aware of your fuel gauge and make sure that you are getting the hydration you need, not just the beverage that's a reflexive go to.

So how are you doing? Zero. Really need to work on your food and water intake. 10! You've got it dialed in. You've mastered it. Moving on.

System 3~ Maintenance.

Remember your maintenance equates to self-care and movement. Are you taking time for yourself? Are you moving your body? Are you in nature? Are you getting out? Are you doing activities you enjoy? Your body needs that.

You may be in a place where you have allergies or you're photosensitive, how have you adapted to meet your body's needs?

I'm really lucky because my lupus is not, for some people sun can be a trigger for their skin, for mine it actually is healing and I've learned that if I'm out for about 20 minutes with as much skin exposed as possible to get that vitamin D influence, because I only get it about three months out of the year where I live. Then I make sure that I'm protecting against the sun if I need to be out in the elements for longer than 20 minutes. That really is a perfect ratio for my body to keep my skin healthy.

Maybe the chemicals you're putting on to protect you from the sun or your skincare/beauty routine is not a healthy thing to put on your skin. Your skin is the biggest organ, right? It absorbs. So, everything you're putting on your skin goes into your blood. Many of the chemicals on your skin equate to your cells like junk food.

That's my radical rule of thumb for anything that goes on my skin, whether it's cosmetics or skincare. Can I eat it? If it's safe enough for me to eat and put in my mouth, then that means it's safe enough for me to put on my skin. Ultimately, it's all going to the same place, my organs, blood, and cells.

So for me, if I can eat it, then I'm going to put it on my skin. If it has questionable ingredients that I'm not going to ingest, or if it says 'for external use only', it's probably not something I want to put on externally either. Ultimately, it's all going to end up internally.

Have you abandoned and forgotten to take time for yourself and are not really moving your body? You're withdrawn and so busy taking care of everybody else that you don't have any time for yourself. So busy working you can't get outside. You know you're in that same hamster wheel routine day after day. That's going to be on the lower end of the scale.

Maybe you've got it figured out! You have and know exactly what your routine looks like. You know how your activities are different by the seasons, what your demands are, what your abilities are, and what your interests are. You know where you want to be, what you want to be doing. Do you want to be hiking a mountain or do you want to be on the beach?

You know, and you've got it dialed in. And, more importantly, you have plans and you're making it happen. Okay, that's the ten.

System 4~ Oil

This is your system for supplements and this also changes seasonally. It should, right? You should not be taking the same supplements day in and day out. That's not what a supplement is.

A supplement is to support areas that need more nutrients. They need a tweaking. For example, in the winter, I don't get enough vitamin D because of where I live and my body doesn't necessarily assimilate it as efficiently as it should because of the damage to my organs.

I will always make sure I supplement vitamin D in the winter. Additionally, I'll usually have some zinc and some vitamin C because I'm around a lot of sick people and I'm indoors a lot more in the winter.

I always have my Juice Plus+® foundation, which is a little bit different because it is food so it's not a true supplement that's isolated or targeting a specific organ or system. I do eat it all of the time, but I do tend to adjust and take more in the winter. Again, if I'm around a lot of sick people, travelling, or if I'm overwhelmed and stressed.

My winter supplementation looks different. I might add in some ashwagandha or some rhodiola, again, depending on my systems and what I'm needing. In the summer, I'm what I would call 'supplement light', because I'm getting more vitamin D from the sun. I'm getting a lot of vitamin C and A and minerals because I'm eating a lot of raw food, and a lot of green leafy vegetables.

So, I don't need as much of the isolated C and D, zinc and, and those kinds of supplements. I also eat a lot of herbs. If I'm getting them fresh, why would I take them in a supplement that is not nearly as effective anyway?

Do you know and understand your supplements? Have you changed them? As you're changing your fuel, you're changing your supplements, right?

Score zero if either you don't supplement at all, or you're just taking what you thought you were supposed to take. You've got your daily multivitamin that you take 365, regardless of how you're feeling or what's going on. That's going to be on the lower end.

If you're adjusting for the seasons. You know what you're taking and why you're taking it. You adjust it based on your body, age, and your lifestyle. That's going to be a 10.

System 5~the driver

The mind and intelligence. This is your learning. This is your belief system. Are you open to the growth? Are you planning? Are you excited? Did you spend your spring cultivating ideas and opportunities? And now in the summer, you're ready to take them on and receive them and fertilize and water and grow those opportunities.

Or are you no different today than yesterday? Tomorrow doesn't matter. Very limiting beliefs, lots of fear and scarcity mentality. I've been there! That was my MO (method of operation). That's where my autoimmune diseases were born. Living in that mindset.

What is the tape you have playing in your head? What is your mind telling you it can or cannot accomplish? What environment are you allowing yourself to be in that is supporting or defeating you? What are you learning? How are you growing?

Rate it zero - 10. Ten is that you are thriving, you've got your dreams by the tail, and shooting for the moon. You know exactly what you're doing, how you're going to get there, and you are thriving. You have an unlimited mindset, and you are going for it!

Note: the mere fact that you are reading this book leads me to believe that you likely are on the higher end of this scale because you are exploring a lifestyle of thriving not surviving!

System 6~ Navigation System

The number six system in the Living WOW Framework is your spirit. That voice of truth, right? Who you were born to be? Who you really are when it's just you in the room. Are you slowing down and listening? Do you trust that voice of truth inside of you?

Or have you been let down and not really sure you can trust? Maybe feeling a bit broken or betrayed by your body. Are you not really sure about the mind, body, spirit connection thing?

Are you listening to your voice of truth? Are you trusting your voice? Zero is down in doubt, not practicing any faith, not believing that you matter, or that you were created for a purpose.

Ten is that you have a daily routine. You have a personal connection with your creator. Your faith is strong and you are living true to who you were born to be. Not necessarily who the world is telling you to be, but who you were born to be.

System 7~ Indicator Lights

Your symptoms or autoimmune conditions are number 7 in the Living WOW framework, because they are that outward manifestation of what's happening on the inside. Are you listening to your symptoms?

For me, it's fatigue. It's my skin. It's my organs. It's pain. The cocktail of symptoms that come with the autoimmune diseases of rheumatoid arthritis, oral lichen planus and systemic lupus. Those are the areas that tend to give me the most indicators.

What are your indicator lights saying to you? Are you in a flare? Are you in crisis? Are you hurting? Are you exhausted? That's going to be at the lower end of zero to ten scale.

Ten is you are thriving. You've got energy. Your conditions are in remission or elimination. They're gone.

System 8~Driving Conditions

This may be the most difficult of all of the systems because you have the least control over the environment around you. Sure, by taking care of the other 7 systems you will be ideally prepared for and able to navigate intentionally through your day.

That's the purpose of Living WOW! Having the framework to make intentional choices throughout your day so that you don't get swept away in the current of the SAD life.

How are you doing in defensive driving through SAD? Are you road raging? Have you taken so many pitstops and detours that you forgot where you're going? Are you white knuckling through the storms of life alone because you forgot to turn on your navigator or open the mind of your driver?

Rate zero – 10 on where you are in your driving conditions right now.

Living WOW
Lifestyle Assessment

Review and rate each of the 8 systems below with 0 being no
awareness or autopilot and 10 being mastery and intentional choices.

System	Rate 0-10
Energy (Batteries & Electrical System)	0 1 2 3 4 5 6 7 8 9 10
Food & Water (Fuel)	0 1 2 3 4 5 6 7 8 9 10
Self Care & Movement (Maintenance)	0 1 2 3 4 5 6 7 8 9 10
Supplements (Oil)	0 1 2 3 4 5 6 7 8 9 10
Mind/Intelligence (Driver)	0 1 2 3 4 5 6 7 8 9 10
Spirit (Navigation System)	0 1 2 3 4 5 6 7 8 9 10
Symptoms (Indicator Lights)	0 1 2 3 4 5 6 7 8 9 10
Environment (Driving Conditions)	0 1 2 3 4 5 6 7 8 9 10

Rank

Results:

**After rating, rank each system 1 being lowest and 8
being the highest.**
Focus on 3 lowest scoring systems ranked 1-3

Now look back at each of your scores and identify the three lowest
scores. What three systems do you have the lowest score in? That's
where you will want to spend your time. Do your deep dive and really
work on those 3 areas.

This is why Living WOW was created. This system of awareness and
review is the secret to thriving. I'm not saying this to be proud or

boastful. I'm saying it because I want you to know you can get there because I've been at zeros in all 8 of these systems throughout my life.

When I'm 5 and under it shows. That's where I end up in dis-ease. On the other hand, when I can be in 6-10, I'm on the upside. I'm making progress. I can feel it. And sometimes it'll slide back down. Then I have to course correct. But, if I know those 8 systems, I can plug in and thrive.

Start here. Where you are.

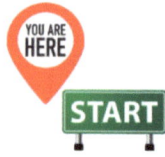

Lifestyle changes can be so overwhelming that most people won't even begin. We rationalize it's not a good time. I have _____ coming up, a holiday, birthday, event. It's too hard. I don't have that kind of willpower. What will people think? My family won't do it.

Unfortunately, in my experience, most people will live in either the River Denial or on Someday Isle until something brings an unpleasant reality and needed perspective at a level of desperation that necessitates a lifestyle change.

I'm no exception. I was living with chronic pain and obesity and didn't even realize how limiting it was because I was just surviving. It was normal. Everyone has pain. Everyone is overweight. Everyone is exhausted. It's part of getting older. Until I had a wakeup call with a bonus baby. I realized that given my family health history, I had a very good chance of having a premature death at worst, or a really crummy quality of life at best.

I realized that this baby deserved to have a mother and her children deserved a grandmother. I had purposely had my children when I was young, ages 22 and 25, because I was the bonus baby who had no living grandparents and a widowed mother when my dad died when I was 16 years old. I had the old parents being the baby by 15, 13, and 9 years.

I believed that if I had my children young, I would beat the odds and be the young parent. My plan worked flawlessly and my health followed the path of my parents until I really followed the path of my parents and had a baby 11 years later when I was 36. As I approached my 40th birthday with a three-year-old, I was desperate to get off Someday Isle and out of the River Denial.

When you're ready, the teacher will appear. This was the beginning of my transformation and ironically the catalyst for change that carried me through my autoimmune journey which you can read about in my book, *8 Lessons Lupus Taught Me: From Surviving to Thriving with Autoimmune Diseases* or on the podcast *Living WOW Out Loud*. (And if you want to meet my bonus baby, she is a guest on episode 10 and now singer/songwriter Jenna Rae ~ Yes! A shameless plug.)

I want to get you out of the river and off of the isle. Don't wait for a crisis.

Unfortunately, so many wait until it's too late, like my dad, and never get a second chance. Use someone else's crisis if you need it for motivation. Use my crisis if you need to. Just get out of the SAD life before it's too late.

So, that sounds very dramatic, but what you're hearing is my passion and absolute knowledge that there is a better way and it is so worth it. It's so much better to have vitality and energy than pain and fatigue. It's so much cheaper to eat whole foods, even the expensive ones, than prescription medications, medical procedures, and surgeries.

Maybe you can't prevent it all, but what if you do? What if you just prevent heart disease or diabetes? What if you can eliminate half of your meds? What if you get to see your grandchildren grow up and can take them to Disneyland and keep up?

Let's say you're ready to give it a go. We're getting off Someday Isle *today*.

Where do you want to start? Well, I say let's start where you are because that's the only way I know. You have to get real with where you are because you can't change something you're not aware of. Step out of the River Denial and take inventory. The best way to measure where you are is with blood work, assessments, weights, and measures.

Honestly, in my opinion, how you feel and taking personal inventory is far more important, but it's not very objective. You can't argue with blood work and assessments, but they can be expensive and intrusive. So many people forego them for an easier at home management of weights and measures.

I don't care where you start, but it is important to know where you are when you do start because it will help you determine what might be the most important WOW system to focus on. It also is very rewarding to look back on how far you have come.

An effective strategy to begin a new behavior and have it become a new habit is to replace it with something else. If you try to just eliminate or change a behavior, it's very difficult, but if you introduce a new behavior in place of the old one, then you're much more successful.

Every time you trigger for the old behavior, you replace it with the new behavior and you do it repeatedly until it becomes the desired effortless behavior. It's then a new pattern. That's momentum.

You crave what you eat. In the beginning, I replaced my vitamin regiment with my Juice Plus+®. (Why vitamins are not effective and whole food nutrition is so much more effective is addressed in systems 2 and 4, so you can refer to that for more detail.)

But if you already have the habit of taking vitamins daily, or maybe even prescription medications, then you can just add Juice Plus+® in, and what happens as a side effect is metabolic programming. Because you are eating more fruits and vegetables, your body recognizes it as fruits and vegetables, and you begin to crave more fruits and vegetables even though it's powdered produce in a capsule.

I've really seen it with more vegetables and I think that's because people tend to naturally eat more fruit because they taste better than vegetables. But in my own personal experience with myself and my family, as well as my clients, I hear all the time that they are craving more whole foods.

That's the easiest way to hack that change so that you're not necessarily having to cut out processed food, but your body will naturally start craving the better whole foods.

Next, to hack the actual foods that you're eating, you have to take inventory and recognize where you are. Do what you will do, and start with the things you like.

Pizza's a big thing in our house. It's my go to meal when I'm tired, if I'm stressed, or if I've had a long day. When my give a damn is busted, I go to pizza. So, the way that I made a substitution was to begin ordering more vegetables on my pizza. I took off the processed meats and put on the fresh vegetables. And just by doing that, pizza's still not a health food, but it's a better choice. I'm getting more whole food and getting less processed food.

Maybe pizza's not your thing. Maybe it's a hamburger. Instead of having just a plain cheeseburger, maybe you start adding more veggies on it. You make sure it has fresh lettuce and tomato, or for you, maybe it's grilled onions or mushrooms.

Maybe for you, it's a lettuce wrap instead of a bun, depending on where you are and how you want to kick it up a notch. My husband, for example, has been eating WOW for a long time now because it's become our normal, but we can still refine. He's working hard to eat less processed grains, so he's using lettuce instead of buns to get more of the produce in and less of the processed carbs.

Look where you're at, maybe it's just adding lettuce and tomato to your burger, or maybe you totally take off the burger and replace it with a grilled portobello mushroom. There are all sorts of different things you can do, but the key is not necessarily *what* you do, but that you *do* it.

Start where you're at and look at a particular meal that you would eat and then figure out how you would tweak that meal, then plan accordingly.

That leads to hack number three, because obviously, I can't make a portobello burger if I don't have any mushrooms. Likewise, I can't make a cheeseburger if I don't have cheese, buns, or burgers.

I have to go to the grocery store, so at that point, I make my choice. Am I going to do SAD or am I going to do WOW? If that's what's in my house and that's what I've already planned, then I've already made that substitution and I'm not just eating a bunch of foreign foods that I can't stand or I've never tried.

Instead, I'm eating my comfort foods and the regular foods that I enjoy, but I've made them a little fresher. I've eliminated the processing. Whether it's taking out a processed meat. Whether it's taking out a processed bread. Whether it's getting away from the dyes and chemicals.

It just depends on where you're at and what it is. Just make a substitution that gets you closer to the earth and farther from the factory with your meal planning.

Which leads me to my final hack for now. Planning ahead. Meal planning and stocking your pantry with whole foods rather than boxes, bags, and cans is ultimately where the change from SAD to WOW occurs.

Realize that different family members may have different substitutions. The key is not to take away everyone's favorite foods, but rather to bring them a little closer to whole real foods.

I found that monthly meal plans with everyone's input makes for a successful WOW menu. When I don't get around to it, even though it's quite normal for us to eat WOW and the house is stocked accordingly, we order that pizza and take out way too often.

Maybe that's just us, but we all notice a difference when we plan a monthly menu together as a family. It's magic. So that's my secret to WOW life. Start where you're at. Take inventory and get real.

Living WOW
Lifestyle Prescription

Now that you understand the 8 systems of your lifestyle you are on the road to becoming the expert in your body. As the expert you know how your lifestyle impacts your health and you know how to assess and triage the systems for support and repair.

System at Risk: Circle 1 area of focus

Energy (Batteries & Electrical System)   **Mind/Intelligence (Driver)**

Food & Water (Fuel)   **Spirit (Navigation System)**

Self Care & Movement (Maintenance)   **Symptoms (Indicator Lights)**

Supplements (Oil)   **Environment (Driving Conditions)**

Rx:

Choose 3 activities that will support this system and create an environment of healing.

Do:_____

Frequency: *x per day, week, month, quarter (circle one)*

Duration: *for*   *minutes, days, weeks (circle one)*

Signature _____

Date _____

Why is it important for you to get out of the SAD life? What's at stake for you if you don't make a change?

I guarantee you it's more than you realize. Consider adding Juice Plus+® as a foundation to your whole food nutrition and to help you get into the whole food metabolic programming. Make small substitutions, adding in more whole foods into the food you already love and eat.

Make the choice at the supermarket by clearing your house of some boxes, bags, and cans, and stocking the pantry, refrigerator, and freezer with more whole foods. Finally, plan ahead using what you've stocked and planned for so that you're having fun enjoying your delicious whole foods and not defaulting to convenient automatic foods.

Top 8 Tools for A Budding Mechanic

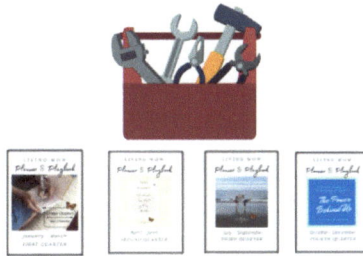

I want to introduce you to some tools for addressing each of the 8 systems, and for the sake of consistency, I will continue to use the vehicle metaphor with you as the mechanic. You are ultimately the one who has the most knowledge about your vehicle. However, you may not be familiar with the variety of tools available to help you clean and maintain your vehicle to have the ultimate driving experience, aka thriving!

Any master mechanic has an organized garage and a system for finding the tool he needs. A specialized toolbox that keeps what is needed available and organized. Accumulating more tools but not knowing where to find them or whether they are even the right type and size for your vehicle is not useful and could be a waste of time and resources making the overwhelming situation of a breakdown even worse.

It is because of this fact that I would be remiss if I didn't first give you a toolbox that can help you find and organize your tools as you accumulate and upgrade them. Over the past 15 years, I have tried many different organization strategies to help me learn, organize, and track these different areas of my lifestyle.

Ultimately, I blended a lifelong organization strategy of a planner and the beneficial activity of journaling with the routine of a daily rhythm. I have talked about these different aspects throughout this book so here is where they all come together into the *Living WOW Planner & Playbook.*

A toolbox of sorts where each of the 8 systems is intentionally integrated to keep you intentional in the daily choices you make and give you the data you need as the master mechanic of your vehicle.

The first half, the *Living WOW Planner* includes a year at a glance, month at a glance, and weekly planner pages that you can plan the big rocks and keep the main thing the main thing and not let outside SAD agendas creep in.

The second half, the *Living WOW Playbook* includes daily pages for a morning Power UP routine that includes movement, study, and meditation with quick assessments and reminders to keep a WOW focus as you launch your day. The evening Power DOWN page is a quick journal to review and report each day as you wind down and restore at the end of the day.

This specialized and robust Planner & Playbook is broken into quarterly editions to keep it manageable and efficient. Earlier versions have been available in digital download, but honestly the printing and organization of it was still asking a lot of you.

In 2025, more cost-effective bound versions are available on Amazon and the CallyRae.com website leaving you more time to use the tools rather than create your toolbox. Check out the website for the current quarter as well as any community promotion that may be happening when you visit!

Living in the modern world with access to information and technology on a continual basis has in many ways tested our confidence as the expert in our bodies. Continuous and often loud or conflicting messages can be overwhelming to tune out and go within to hear and feel what your body is saying to you.

The assessment questions I introduced earlier can be paired with these tools to plug in, practice, and develop mastery as you fine tune your vehicle. Recognize that this is an ongoing process and resist the urge to get frustrated or feel like you are not doing it right.

Remember that you are innately designed for this journey.

Just like you advanced from the passenger as a child to the driver as a teenager, your understanding and skills of your vehicle and journey have continued to refine and learn throughout the rest of your life. If you don't understand all of the nuances of the 8 systems immediately, that's normal. It's not that you can't. Find the modality that works best for you and refine it.

You will likely find that as you become more comfortable and skilled, opportunities will present themselves for you to go deeper, learn more, and heal more. Life has a funny way of providing opportunities for you to learn. Recognizing and showing up to learn is the hard part. I guarantee if you show up, your body will reciprocate and you will thrive as the expert in your body.

Although this list is not comprehensive, it is foundational and powerful. I specifically chose the modalities that are powerful, easy, accessible, and possibly already familiar to you. Again, don't feel like you have to use them all. Start with one or two and explore to see how it connects for you. Just like you have a favorite teacher in school, you'll likely find that you have preferred tools.

As your skills or needs change, you may choose a different tool that you aren't ready for today. Here are my top eight system tools.

Number 1 is breathwork. In my opinion, the most powerful tool for thriving is breathwork. The reason is because you can tune into your breath to get a real time reading of the interactions of your mind, body, and spirit.

In the beginning, it may only be the obvious stress response with shallow or rapid breathing. You can acknowledge and change that response by intentionally deepening or slowing the breath. With practice, you can learn to connect with your spirit through breathwork and use it to bring healing to specific areas of your body or release imbalances or interruptions in your energy fields.

Breathwork is the most powerful way to connect the body to the interplay of the mind and body. Think of it as your internal search engine that can provide you the quickest information and results in real time, anytime, anywhere. Your breath is always with you.

Number 2 is meditation. Probably the best-known modality for healing by creating the quiet space within to experience the mind body connection. Meditation is an essential tool for the body. Taking intentional time to go within and cultivate awareness free of expectation and judgment is a process.

That process will lead you closer to mastery of your 8 systems. Meditation also has expectation and stigma with it. It can feel like the enormous library you walk into to find an answer, but can easily get distracted by volumes of information and how to find or recognize the information that may be in the back of the room or on the top shelf.

Resist the urge to feel like you don't have time, that you can't do it because your mind wanders, or even just feeling like you don't know how. Those are all normal, and the truth is, taking even a minute to close your eyes, breathe, and observe will increase your intention and awareness of your vehicle.

For me, guided meditations help me stay focused. There are many recordings and apps that you can choose and grow your meditation skills with. Explore different types of meditation and integration until you find one that suits you.

Number 3 is tapping or EFT which is the Emotional Freedom Technique. It's great for getting into the body because it utilizes physical touch and the meridians of the body, stimulating and releasing trapped emotions, thoughts, or beliefs helping you to process them.

There are specific techniques for tapping that have been researched to maximize the connection and benefit for finding, metabolizing, and healing trapped beliefs or experiences. With that said, learning the basics of the tapping points, recognizing how you're feeling, and then initiating that communication with your body are the essentials and can be beneficial even at a basic level.

I would recommend using a practitioner in EFT to guide you through the process if you are processing traumatic experiences and emotions. If you're using tapping as a maintenance tool for your lifestyle, you can absolutely learn to do tapping on your own and will find it to be a quick and easy way to reset your energies when you're feeling off.

Tapping can also be powerful in the morning to set your intentions for the day, or in the evening to release and let go of the day's events so that you can rest and recover during sleep. Although you may feel like a silly monkey in the beginning, tapping is a powerful and simple tool that can be a fantastic starting point as the expert in your body.

My favorite is the Tapping Solution, which is available as a book, film, or app. They also host an annual Tapping Summit bringing together many EFT practitioners online for you to learn and apply guided tapping.

Number 4 is massage. The most passive and time-consuming tool is massage. Not all massage is created equal, and you may not have thought of it as a way to maximize understanding of your body. But it absolutely can be a powerful tool, especially when you pair it with breath work and meditation.

A trained practitioner is doing the physical work of massage, but you are in a quiet and often beautiful space during a massage. It's an opportunity for you to notice the physical messages of your body and take inventory of your systems.

You may recognize patterns of pain, knots, weakness, or tenderness that can help you recognize how your body is processing, or not, experiences you've had in the recent days or weeks. Remember that your body is speaking to you with these physical symptoms. Do not ignore your best friend and this opportunity to have a quality intimate conversation during this uninterrupted time.

Number 5 five is yoga. Because of the autoimmune diseases I lived with, the symptoms I experienced resulted in chronic pain throughout my body every day. Yoga became a vital part of my morning routine and was one of my first tools that helped me better understand and trust my body.

As a part of the morning power up routine, it provides a time to stretch and balance your body, tuning in to what is working and what isn't. It increases your capacity to feel and learn where you store your stress, insecurities, fears, and doubts.

Yoga is a gentle and individual way to listen to your body and provide the movement that supports, facilitates, and heals. It allows your body to hear and interpret what your spirit is telling you and where your mind might be limiting you. It may help you recognize where your mind and spirit are at odds.

Number 6 is Qigong or Tai Chi. Similar to yoga, but not as commonly practiced in the United States are Qigong and Tai Chi. I say similar to yoga in that they are body movement practices that have ancient origins for synchronizing breath and movements to understand and heal the spirit, qi, or life force.

These ancient practices have spiritual, medical, and martial branches. I've not spent as much time in the study or practice of the chi art forms, but have enjoyed and benefited from some video trainings and articles about them.

Like yoga, I find them to be gentle on my body and supportive to both my mind and spirit. This is a great environment to practice and develop your expert mechanic skills.

Number 7 energy hygiene is probably the most woo woo of this list because it has the least tangible or physical interaction. Visualizing a ball of light coming in through your crown, flowing through your central channel, and rooting you deep into the earth may sound very foreign to you.

Understanding chakras, auras, grids, and fields are becoming more mainstream with advancing quantum physics and energy measuring devices. However, they remain generally misunderstood and avoided. With that said, you are familiar with how energy feels and as such can understand the need to clear it and repair it, even if you can't see it or understand it.

An example is the person who always has drama and angst that makes you feel tense when they walk into the room. In contrast, the calming energy of a walk through the woods or along the water. Whether you realize it or not, you are picking up those energies and taking a bit of that with you throughout your day.

The status of your energy greatly impacts what you pick up, how long you carry it with you, and how you pass it on. I call these micro energy clearing sessions and I often infuse them into my shower routine. Cleaning the outside of the body is a good time to clean the inside of the body. Dry brushing is also a popular technique that has both physical and energetic benefits.

Some of the energy workers that I have learned from are Donna Eden, Dr. Andrew Weil, and Carol Tuttle.

Number 8 is AMA bodywork or reflexology. Both of these interpreters use trigger points, organ systems, and the meridians to access the energy centers through physical touch and manipulation. Skilled practitioners can identify and help you understand your body language by identifying where energetic leaks or injuries are present.

Much like massage, once you identify what your body needs, you can support it with deeper conversation to create the environment to heal. In the beginning, I used external experts and interpreters to help me move my energy because I didn't understand and recognize body language.

As I have become more and more fluent in body language, I'm now able to recognize and have daily conversations with my body all the time, just like I have conversations with people all the time.

I understand that when my body gives me a symptom, I look at what has just happened in my beliefs, in my energy, and in my circumstances. I'm able to interpret that external manifestation as understanding what my body is telling me. A common thread among all these interpreters is taking time and quieting the world around you for just a moment to listen and communicate with your body.

The level of communication will change as your understanding grows. I have found a structured routine to be beneficial to prioritize the 8 systems. Starting with bookends of the day ensures that there is time and space to be intentional.

My ideal Power Up is 20 minutes of movement, 20 minutes of study, and 20 minutes of meditation. It took years to cultivate, and some mornings, it doesn't look like that at all. But when it does, I'm at my best, and it's worth it.

This is an excellent time and place to assess your 8 systems. Set the intentions for the day. Get your beliefs and physical body in the same conversation. You may get started with one tool to help you understand your body language during this time and eventually find yourself exploring different modalities to expand your understanding.

Power Down evening routine is powerful for sleep hygiene and a great opportunity to take inventory of the day.

My ideal power down is the hour prior to lights out and includes 20 minutes of review, 20 minutes of report, and 20 minutes of restore. Inventory is a natural time to initiate reflection and gratitude as you check in to see how the systems are functioning and progressing. This may include journaling, meditation, gratitude, and prayer.

Not sure what to ask? Pick up with where you left off in the morning with the conversation starters and intentions. It's important to have a space that is quiet and restorative to power down. You don't want to be shouting at your body amid the television shows or social media conversations.

If you're having a hard time winding down, I highly recommend tapping as a go to tool to help release the chaos of the day and set a new rhythm to rest and restore.

The disclaimer: none of these tools will cause you any harm, no side effects or damage. There is no level of expertise you have to have in order to explore and learn these tools. Go at the pace you want and find the modality that works best for you. It takes time to develop efficiency in these tools like it does in any new skill.

I promise you that it is so worth it. I promise you that you are capable of it. I promise you that you are the expert in your body. You will be able to listen and understand your body in the midst of all the chaos and distraction of the world around you. You can create the environment to thrive living WOW as you systematically and intentionally step away from living SAD.

About The Author

CallyRae is best known for her professional accomplishments as a Speech Language Pathologist and her specialized treatment of tongue thrust as the creator and author of the *Stone Tongue Thrust Protocol: A Protocol for the Assessment and Treatment of Tongue Thrust*. She gets satisfaction out of telling her childhood teachers that she found a way to make her "talking too much in class" pay off. Now she not only gets paid for talking but also for teaching others to do the same.

Through her transformation journey with Autoimmune Diseases, CallyRae found another passion of inspiring healthy living. She has become an author, speaker, transformation coach, certified nutritionist, podcaster, and now lifestyle engineer advocating and educating about the power of lifestyle choices. Her passion of inspiring hope where there is hopelessness, confidence where there is fear, and joy where there is sadness has led her to create the Living WOW Lifestyle as a system to thrive regardless of your circumstance or diagnosis.

As an insatiable lifelong learner, CallyRae is innovative and eclectic. She loves to encourage and educate people about their potential and give them the tools to strive for more. She seems to gravitate to the challenges and seek for the solution. She believes in the Divine and miraculous and rejects the reasonable and practical believing that everyone has the right to live their best life.

CallyRae is the proud mother and grandmother of Jessica, Christopher, Jenna, and Mikayla (with hopefully more to come). She is married to her best friend and companion, Joff.

She loves to travel and experience new places, but the best part is always coming back home and spending time with family. Her perfect day would be on a beach or on the road creating content to educate, inspire, and empower you to embrace who you were born to be and live your best life.

OTHER RESOURCES BY *CallyRae:*

You can follow CallyRae on her website *CallyRae.com* for information and links to her latest creations, content, and social media for thriving and Living WOW.

Living WOW Out Loud: Thriving with Autoimmune Diseases podcast available wherever you listen

Living WOW Planner & Playbook updated quarterly and available on the website or Amazon

8 Lessons Lupus Taught Me: From Surviving to Thriving with Autoimmune Diseases available in print, eBook, and audio book

Change Your Story: From Surviving to Thriving with Autoimmune Diseases Presentation available on You Tube

www.ingramcontent.com/pod-product-compliance
Lightning Source LLC
Chambersburg PA
CBHW042128080426
42735CB00001B/5